The Natural Hair Bible

THE 10 COMMANDMENTS OF BLACK HAIR CARE

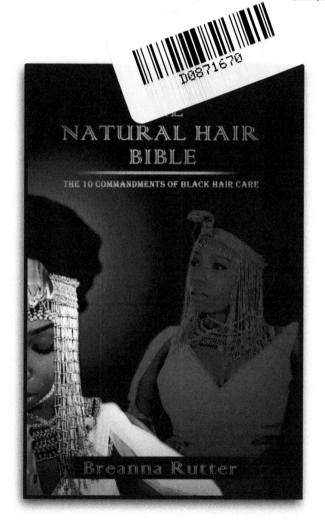

HOWTOBLACKHAIR LLC.

WRITTEN BY AUTHOR BREANNA RUTTER

TABLE OF CONTENTS

THE AUTHOR'S STORY

Before I begin to go into detail and paint the picture of my hair story, I first want to talk a little bit about what finally led me to becoming an author. Being an author is not something that I had seen in my future or had hopes for. Being an author is not the dreams girls dreamt coming from where I am from.

I was born and raised during the most precious moments of my childhood on the south side of Chicago Illinois. It was not all bad and it was not all good from what I could remember, and that is probably because every child is naive of the world they live in until they start to grasp their world. As a kid I hated being naïve and that drove me to ask questions, I wanted to know it all!

I was never a smart alec and I always hated being told, "you're too young" or "wait until you're older" to receive knowledge that I was asking for. Not knowing things turned me into a hard core knowledge seeking investigator because I had come to the conclusion that if you want to know something, you have to figure it out yourself. Maybe that was not the intent behind the answer my parents gave me but that is how I perceived the answers to my questions when they went unanswered.

Writing was something I never knew I really had a passion for until I started to pay attention to this area of my creativity. In class, I always volunteered to read out loud or volunteered to peer edit the papers of my classmates and of course the extra credit was definitely a bonus! There were times when I would get a B or C letter grade on my paper and that would baffle me. This did not come from a place of entitlement to receive an A because of my confidence in writing; it came from my inner desire to question everything that I did not understand. When I poured my heart and soul into every research paper that I had slaved over for weeks or months at a time, I wanted to know why I did not ace it. Why was my paper credited a C? Did I have a lot of spelling errors? Did I forget to properly indent the first sentence of every paragraph, or was I negligent to credit my resources in my references section? Did I correctly punctuate? Could you guess the answers I received time and time again from various teachers throughout elementary school, high school, and onto college? You copied or you cheated, the way things were written looks as if you copied some of your writing from someone word for word. Who could I have possibly cheated from and how could I have remained consistent in my writing abilities throughout years of schooling? My writing and reading capabilities were always at the top of my class, actually at least two grades ahead. I always had to rewrite my rough drafts and write sample essays for my English teachers to prove that my writing capabilities were truthfully mine. This saddened me to always be doubted and then it made me feel proud in the same breath because I know for a fact that everything that I had written in that very paper was from my own writing capabilities and when my English teachers read it, they often would refuse to believe I didn't cheat in some type of way. It honestly became the highest form of flattery to me especially when I doubted myself time and time again in my writing capabilities. I would like to thank my favorite English teacher, Mrs. Fitch, for seeing the vision of me being an author before I could see it for myself; you will always have a special place in my heart.

Similarly, I have gone through a like experience in regards to my ability to do my hair or anyone else's hair. The first time anyone had ever doubted me with hair was when I braided my mother's hair in micro braids. It probably took me about three days to finish her entire head because I wasn't used to standing for hours like a typical braider and also because I had chores, school, and homework to do every day as well. I braided enough braids around the perimeter of her head so that she could wear her hair to work in a high bun. When she came back from work she bought a friend with her who wanted to see first-hand my braiding skills. I didn't mind because everyone assumed that I was too young to know how to braid well. The thing that bothered me about this was that this woman was a total stranger to me and she felt comfortable enough to critique me and hang over my shoulder when she doesn't know how to braid hair! What surprised me was to hear her say that I was good, but too young to do someone's hair. How rude!

Out of many similar experiences, another that really stood out to me was when I was a junior in high school. The color of my hair was honey blonde box dyed with dark brown roots. I had an extreme side part sew in with long wavy hair that stopped above my waist and I also had cornrow designs on the side of my head. The hair style was very beautiful and different from everyone else's hair at the time. Everyone at school was going through the Nicki phase, wearing jet black hair with Chinese bangs and I refused to wear my hair how everyone else had worn theirs. For the life of my hairstyle that I had worn, someone would come up to me almost every day at school and ask who did my hair and if that person could do their hair similar to mine. I always said the same thing and I would get the same answer, I would say,

"I did this style, I do my own hair and I could do your hair if you like."

The same rely was, "Oh you did, well never mind..."

Never mind?!? I assumed that people did not believe me for whatever reason or just did not want me to do their hair. I rarely received compliments for my ability to do my own hair but my peers always complimented me on how flattering my hairstyles were. Why was it so hard for people to believe that I had the ability to do my own hair that well? Another person had even walked up to me while I was still wearing the same hairstyle and asked me who did my hair, I said "I did" and before I could say anything else, they stormed off and said,

"Wow, you're lying, you didn't do that!"

This happened all the time while I was in high school no matter what hairstyle I would wear. Being that I did not have much, and that every dollar at home had to stretch, I had to shop at the thrift store to buy affordable clothes. With any money I would make from braiding my friend's hair, I would make sure to use that money to wear very flattering hairstyles because I knew that made up for any lack I may have had. My hair definitely did just that, no one ever brought up the fact that I was wearing the same winter boots every school year or that I only had a couple of pairs of jeans. No one ever said anything about the plain shoulder sling backpack that I would wear to school; anyone that would ever approach me at school was mesmerized by my hair.

After graduating high school, the interaction I received about my hair was different. For instance, just a couple of months ago, I stopped into my local beauty supply store just to pick up some hair oils that I was running low on and someone asked me about my box braids. They wanted to know who did them and the cost and when I told them I did, they wanted me to do their hair as soon as I was available! There were also some girls in the store, who I had never seen before, confess that they thought I had the prettiest hair in school and that they always wanted to know who did my hair and when I told them I did, they wanted me to do their hair too!

I started realizing back in high school that I had a talent. All the practice that went into perfecting my hairstyles was well worth it and admired by many. From my own personal experiences, I've encountered many people who did not know how to do hair well and they had an even harder time doing their own hair. I thought that it would be a good idea to share my techniques and tips on video and upload them to YouTube to share with them and others. I am glad that I did because the amounts of responses that I receive from my YouTube tutorials have been so positively overwhelming! Every day I receive countless email messages, video, Facebook, and Twitter comments about how helpful my hairstyling videos are and how much it helped them in their ability to do their own hair. After publishing hundreds of hair tutorials to my YouTube channel, seeing is definitely believing because now I hardly ever receive doubt from others!

I've walked these parts of my life to say this, the things that you are good at will seem impossible for you to separate yourself from. It will always draw you back in to remind you that you just can't run away no matter how long or fast you have been running.

Writing has always been within me and I always doubted the chance of being an author because I did not go to school for it and English teachers would often discredit my honesty frequently on papers that I would work so hard on. From this, I realized that the dream and vision you see for yourself is not seen by those around you. They weren't born with what you were born with nor should you expect them to receive that revelation about you. I pursued what was set on my heart, regardless of external pressures, and now I am proud to produce a book for you on a passion that has a strong hold on me since I was a little girl, hair.

Hair was always been the highlight of my life ever since I was a little girl. Getting my hair styled for moments like birthday parties, graduation ceremonies, and holidays spent with family, amongst other examples as well, was the moment I would feel most pretty and sometimes the moment where the pain of styling made me want to shave my head bald just so I didn't have to get my hair done. Trust me; I actually pondered the thought of buzzing my head right before it was time for another relaxer touchup!

One of the most horrible experiences that I could remember with relaxers was when I scratched my head all day forgetting that I had to have a relaxer touch up on my roots the next day. I wanted to cry because I already had eczema on my scalp and I knew that it would not end well! Without the creamy crack (the slang name for a relaxer), I refused to take school pictures. So guess what, on top of an inflamed scalp, the relaxer burned me so bad, I had to rinse my scalp immediately with ice cold water because cold water was the only way I could relieve the burn from my relaxer treatments. I probably had the relaxer on my head for about five minutes so I had extremely puffy roots with straight ends and the right side of my head had a dime sized bald spot of hair missing from traces of relaxer not being properly rinsed off. From my school pictures, everything worked out just fine but that was a relaxer experience that I will never forget or relive again!

Another hair experience I had, come from the ability of not being able to do my own hair. At the time, my mother was working two jobs while my step father was a stay at home parent to my two younger sibling brothers and I. As usual, my mother would go off to work before we came home from school but this time, she had to work overtime. She did not tell my step father about this because it had slipped her mind and on the previous day, she told me to take down my braids and wash my hair so that she could style my hair into a ponytail for me for school the next day. The next day comes and my hair looked like "who did it and what for"? To my demise, my mother was not home, waiting for me in her work clothes, at the kitchen table with an old popcorn tin filled with hair accessories, a hair brush, a warm cup of water, and that infamous blue hair grease. I started crying because I hated going to school without my hair combed and my grandmother wasn't there that morning to help me either.

My last straw of hope was asking my stepfather to fix my hair. He had no idea what to do or how to do it and we both knew it. I told him to just try to do it exactly how mom does it with various materials and I'm quite sure it probably sounded like rocket science to him. I had no idea what he was doing on top of my head and I don't think he did either. I looked in the mirror and wanted to hide under a rock because traces of black hair jel were dried on the back of my neck and my body heat was causing my hairline to look extremely greasy because he used hair grease on my hair. My hair doesn't stop education so I pretty much had no choice but to go to school. My hair at school that day was so hard, you could knock on it and it would sound like a door knock! Also my ponytail was so shrunken because the ponytail wasn't done tight enough on top of unrelaxed new growth!

Both of these hair stories are a horror inside of me that I never will relive again. If these things did not happen, I probably would have never made the decision to go natural, say no to relaxers, or even learn how to do my own hair. As much as I wished these things never happened to me, because of the pain and embarrassment that it caused, looking back today, I know that if I didn't experience this, I wouldn't be writing you this very book today. This book will always be an inspiration to me and hopefully to you as well as you travel on your hair journey.

THE INTRODUCTION TO THE NATURAL HAIR BIBLE

This book is about the basic knowledge that you need to know if you are still pondering the thought of going natural or, you have decided to go natural but you need a help book that you can use as a reference. If you are relaxed, going natural is usually not an easy step to take because your entire hair care practice has to be reevaluated and a new one has to be set in place. Being that going natural changes some aspect of your lifestyle, in regards to your hair, this discourages many from deciding to take that step in their hair journey because they are either comfortable, don't feel the need to, or has a worry for how others will perceive them. Of course you can still maintain healthy hair if you do continue to use relaxers but this book is intended for those who want to know how to take care of their natural hair and/or is in need of encouragement and motivation.

The first commandment of The Natural Hair Bible will start by addressing the idea of worshipping other hair types. Through this commandment, this book will help you to understand the hair typing system as well as how to acquire a different curl pattern.

For the second commandment, this book will talk about fleeing from relaxers, texturizers, and heat. This book will discuss the topic of heat training your hair instead of relaxing your hair and also, in this commandment, the discussion will be opened up about your reason behind relaxing your hair.

In the third commandment, this book will thoroughly talk about why it is so important to cut your damaged ends. Within the black hair community, many women in particular hang on to every strand of hair because when you cut it, they think that it will never grow back. This book will address how untrue that reasoning is and also, talk on natural hair damage and what dry hair really means.

In the fourth commandment, this book will address the importance of the relationship between healthy black hair and water. Black hair (ethnic hair) is usually the driest of hair types and a false taboo is that frequently wetting of the hair is not appropriate. This commandment will help you to see how direct the correlation is between water and constant dry hair. Also, this commandment will discuss the topic of refreshing your curls and swimming with natural hair as well.

The fifth commandment will elaborate on the importance of using natural ingredients in your hair care products. This commandment will not focus on what people think are natural products or not, this commandment will give you great suggestions on homemade recipes that you can use to care for your hair. This commandment will also give you guides as to what ingredients you should make sure to stay away from in your hair care products as well.

The sixth commandment is about the naïve world of being a natural hair nazi. This commandment will discuss the extreme take on hair products, hair extensions, and curl patterns when it comes to natural hair. It is always best to take someone's extreme stance on any topic with a grain of salt because if you want to have a successful natural hair journey, being extreme can complicate what may seem to be an already complicated situation.

In the seventh commandment, the entire discussion will be all about weaves. The previous commandment went into the ideology about weave/extensions and this commandment will help you to embrace them if you so choose to. This commandment will showcase pictures of various hairstyles that can be achieved on natural hair and tutorial suggestions that you can watch to learn how to do them step by step with a plethora of details.

The eighth commandment will discuss how to address "aggressive creamy crack individuals" and also how to be encouraging and not demeaning to others when it comes to the topic of hair. Not everyone will view your hair the same as you and this commandment will highlight the hostility between those who choose to relax their hair and those who choose to wear their hair in its natural state. Also, this book will discuss how to encourage those who are seeking encouragement when it comes to natural hair and, how to respond to the ignorance or hate of others without being demeaning.

In the ninth commandment, I will walk you step by step on how to maintain the health of your hair, by developing a hair care routine. This commandment will go in the natural order that you would normally care for your hair in the order provided;

detangling, conditioner washing, shampooing, deep conditioning, moisturizing and protective styling.

In the tenth commandment, above all else, learn to love and accept your own hair. When choosing to wear your hair in its natural state, you still want it to reflect your lifestyle so this hair bible will help you to understand how to do what works for you. The psychological aspects of black hair will also be unearthed because it is not talked about enough nor are we recognizing its impact. We will learn how to overcome the scars and begin to heal from our personal experiences, and the stigmas associated with natural hair. Also, to big chop or not to big chop does not have to be that devastating fork in the road between choosing to embrace your natural hair, or continuing to cling on to your relaxed hair. And finally, we will listen to ourselves and our hair. You live with what's on top of your head before anyone else does, so it's time to listen to yourself and your hair because the decision is ultimately yours. You are living your life so live it how you choose.

COMMANDMENT I

DO NOT WORSHIP OTHER HAIR TYPES

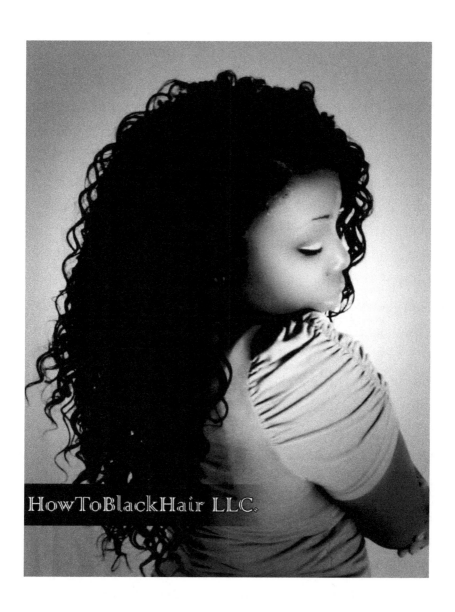

INTRODUCTION TO COMMANDMENT I

BEING THAT I AM IN MY 20'S

Being that I am in my 20's, there is a small pool of natural haired women, of a similar age group, who are idolized for their tresses. In this day and age, it is normal to see majority of women sporting either a weave or extension hairstyle because in the society we live in, it is normal or for lack of better word, deemed "more acceptable" to wear a weave instead of your natural hair. Back in the day, let's say between the 60's and 80's era, afros and jheri curls were in full effect! Recently my mother and I were talking about hair and she took me back in the day, down her memory lane, when she would wear her hair in jheri curls, she thought it was so hot! Of course she laughed off that moment in her life and said that she won't bring it up again. She even said I will never find a picture because she destroyed them all, no one will ever see her greasy forehead photos with jheri curl juice dripping down her neck! That tickled me pink because we all have been there through an embarrassing hair phase. When you go through life's phases, so will your hair.

Today, my age crowd within the natural hair world drools over celebrities like Solange Knowles, Elle Varner, Chisette Michele, Tracee Ross, Esperanza Spalding and Janelle Monae, just to name a few. All the ladies mentioned above are beautiful, cool, and funky in their own ways. Shamelessly wearing their natural hair adds a depth to how they choose to portray themselves to the world because you can't blend in with the rest when being you. Some women mentioned above have very tight curl patterns while some have looser curl patterns and both types are idolized by many. This can be unhealthy when you hair looks nothing like your idol's but it can also be healthy if their hair looks very similar to yours. This can give you a realistic expectation of how particular hair types look at long and short lengths. Please remember to keep in mind that their hair is not your hair no matter how similar it looks to yours. The same goes for a product that a celebrity might use. On her hair, the products can absorb beautifully while in your case, it sits on top of your strands, flakes up, and becomes of no good for you. The go home point is to have no expectation of what your hair will look like and to accept whatever grows out of your head, this will save you from much heartache and disappointment.

THE HAIR TYPING SYSTEM

The hair typing system is either encouraged or discouraged within the natural hair community. It is discouraged by some because it can bring divide between curly individuals, and it is encouraged by some because it provides insight to know which products would be helpful over others when it comes to various hair types. For example, the tighter your curl pattern is, the more appreciative your hair will be towards heavier hair creams and butters. The looser your curl pattern, the better your hair will appreciate creams and moisturizers. In this commandment, two popular hair typing systems will be addressed such as the LOIS Hair Typing System and the Andre Walker Hair Typing System.

THE LOIS HAIR TYPING SYSTEM

The LOIS Hair Typing System demonstrates the shape of your hair strands with the shape of its letters representing the shape of your strands. Also the LOIS System gives a break down not only of your hair type but also of your hair texture according to its feel and absorbency. The LOIS Hair Typing System has existed before the Andre Walker Hair Typing System so it is only fitting to begin with LOIS first.

When figuring out where your hair lies in regards to the LOIS system, you should have freshly washed and naturally dried hair for an accurate finding of your hair type/curl pattern. Using clean shed hair after detangling your hair would be fitting as well. Make sure that your hair dries without taking on the form of a manipulated hairstyle.

- L — Your hair will sharply bend at angles. Your strands bend like the shape of this letter. You will have little to no curves in your hair strands. Your hair type is L.

- O — Your hair has a continuous spiral from the roots to the ends. Think of the shape of a slinky toy. Your hair type is O.

- I — Your hair is straight and lies flat. You have no bends or curves. Your hair type is I.

- S — Your hair will have a loose and/or tight wave pattern. This type does not look like L or O; you will see waves, not bends (L type) or coils (O type). Your hair type is S.

It is natural if your hair fits different hair types so just take on the most dominate hair type as your own. If it is hard to decide between your two most dominant choices, combine them (IL type, OS type, so on and so forth).

Now that you have figured out your hair type, the same hair conditions will apply to understanding the texture of your hair.

Understanding the texture of your hair will prepare you to understand your hair needs even further. You should have freshly washed and naturally dried hair for an accurate finding of your texture. Make sure that your hair dries without taking on the form of a manipulated hairstyle. Also, to help you to understand the difference between shine and sheen, remember that hair with sheen has a low luster glow and hair with shine projects a strong shiny reflection.

The LOIS System for hair textures go as follow;

- Thready — This hair texture has a low sheen and a high shine if the hair is held taut; like in braids or twists. This hair texture has low frizz, wets easily, but water dries out quickly.

- Wiry —This hair texture has a sparkly sheen, with low shine and low frizz. Water beads up or bounces off the hair strands. This hair never seems to get fully wet.

- Cottony — This hair texture has a low sheen, a high shine if held taut, and has high frizz. This hair absorbs water quickly but does not feel thoroughly wet very fast.

- Spongy — This hair texture has a high sheen and low shine with a compacted looking frizz. This hair absorbs water quickly before it feels thoroughly wet.

- Silky — This hair texture has low sheen, a very high shine, with a lot or low frizz. This hair type easily wets in water.

Now that you have decided your hair type and texture, your hair texture will help you to determine your level of moisture needs. Black hair tends to be the driest of hair types so across the board of hair textures, you will need to use sealants (oils) to from a barrier around your wet strands. Oil seals water into your hair for your moisture needs.

- Thready

This hair texture wets easily so locking in moisture with light oils are appropriate. Using light oils like coconut oil and jojoba oil are ideal. Serums add shine and since thready hair has a nice shine when held taut in styles, serums are not a necessity. Also, because this hair texture has low frizz, using glycerin in humid environments can keep your strands plump and juicy without resulting in a frizz. Even though your hair is thready, that does not mean that your hair is typical. Use this as a guide while also experimenting to see what products/ingredients will work for you.

- Wiry

This hair texture has low shine so the use of light to heavy serums will give you the shine that you crave since you have a lack thereof. This hair type also slowly retains and releases moisture based off of its moisture needs so using light to semi-heavy oils like coconut oil, jojoba oil, and olive oil would be best. Even though your hair is wiry, that does not mean that you hair is typical. Use this as a guide while also experimenting to see what products/ingredients will work for you.

- Cottony

This hair texture has more shine than sheen which means that your hair type is always in need of water (moisture). Because of this, your hair type will absorb water quickly, expanding in size, before your hair actually feels wet to touch. Also this hair texture has the most frizz so stay away from humectants like honey and glycerin. If you still want to test out humectants, use humectants in small amounts. Keeping your hair moisturized with this hair texture will result in the optimum health of this hair type, so heavier hair creams, butters, and oils are usually best. Choose options like olive oil, Shea butter, cocoa butter, and grape seed oil, just to name a few, to lock water into your strands. Even though your hair is cottony, that does not mean that you hair is typical. Use this as a guide while also experimenting to see what products/ingredients will work for you.

- Spongy

This hair texture has similar behavior qualities as the cottony hair texture but it has high shine and low sheen while the cottony hair texture has opposite. Because this hair tends to be shiny when taut, serums aren't needed unless your hairstyle has little to no tension; like wearing an afro. Naturally, this hair texture can look frizzy and humectants will only encourage more frizz. Use oils to seal in moisture similar to the cottony hair texture. Even though your hair is spongy, that does not mean that you hair is typical. Use this as a guide while also experimenting to see what products/ingredients will work for you.

- Silky

This hair texture absorbs water easily and because of this, heavy butters, oils, and serums will only make the hair feel greasy and weighed down. With easily wetted hair types, little and light product is best. As you may have assumed, little use of light oils such as jojoba and coconut oil would be best, try tea tree oil as well. Serums are not necessary because this hair texture has high shine. Low frizz with this hair texture also means that using humectants will enhance the look of this hair in styles. Even though your hair is silky, that does not mean that you hair is typical. Use this as a guide while also experimenting to see what products/ingredients will work for you.

The LOIS Hair Typing System is a great hair system to use when you want to use hair textures to point you to the products that will best work for your hair. The Andre Walker Hair Typing System is the most recognized hair typing system even though it was invented in the latter. With this hair typing system, your hair care product suggestions rely more on the look of certain curl types

/patterns rather than certain hair textures. Remember, The Andre Walker Hair Typing System relays information based off look while the LOIS Hair Typing System relays information based of texture. Both hair typing systems are very helpful but since the Andre Hair Typing System is infamous with hair typing, let us discover another way to determine your hair type.

THE ANDRE WALKER HAIR TYPING SYSTEM

The Andre Walker Hair Typing System is based off of the look of a curl pattern more than the feel and texture of the curl pattern. The type of curl pattern you have can help you to develop a hair care routine and hair care arsenal. The organization of curl type ranges from numbers 1-4 and letters A-C. The numbers represent the shape of your curl and the letters represent the degree of looseness and /or tightness within that numbered category.

When figuring out where your hair lies in regards to the Andre Walker Hair Typing System you should have freshly washed and naturally dried hair for an accurate finding of your curl pattern. Using clean shed hair after detangling your hair would be fitting as well. Make sure that your hair dries without taking on the form of a manipulated hairstyle.

Curl Pattern 1 - This curl pattern is straight when wet and dry, no curves or bends. That is why Curl Pattern 1 does not have a lettered degree to represent variations within this hair pattern.

Curl Pattern 2 — This curl pattern includes 2A, 2B, and 2C.

This curl pattern varies from slightly wavy to extremely wavy. In relation to hair extensions, your curl pattern will similarly represent a Body Wave (2A), French Wave (2B), or a Deep Ripple (2C).

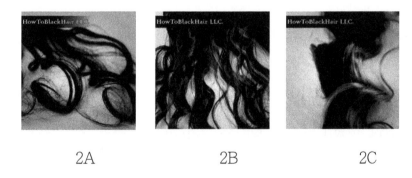

| 2A | 2B | 2C |

If you have more than one dominant curl pattern, choose to take on the pattern that you feel best represents your head of hair.

Curl Pattern 3 - This curl pattern includes 3A, 3B, and 3C.

This curl pattern varies from slightly curly to extremely curly. In relation to hair extensions, your curl pattern will similarly represent a Virgin Indian Curly (3A), Deep Wave (3B), or a Corkscrew Curl (3C)

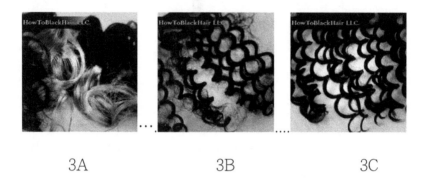

3A   3B   3C

If you have more than one dominant curl pattern, choose to take on the pattern that you feel best represents your head of hair.

Curl Pattern 4 - This curl pattern includes 4A, 4B, and 4C.

This curl pattern varies from zigzagged to coily curl patterns.

In relation to hair extensions, your curl pattern will similarly represent a Jheri Curl (4A), Bohemian Curl (4B), or Afro Kinky (4C).

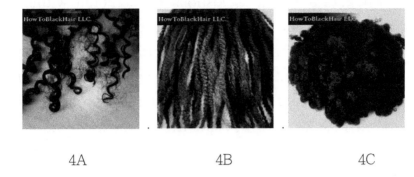

4A   4B   4C

If you have more than one dominant curl pattern, choose to take on the pattern that you feel best represents your head of hair.

Understanding your hair type/texture is important because this understanding will reveal to you how to work with your hair and its conditions. Knowing your curl pattern is also important because you can use curl patterns to relate your hair needs to another who shares similar hair qualities. The reason why it always feels like you hit that same brick wall when it comes to caring for your hair, if it so applies, is because of your lack of knowledge and maybe your own stubbornness, usually caused by frustration. If you know that you have 4C hair according to the Andre Walker Hair Typing System, you will most likely have the cottony or spongy hair texture according to the LOIS Hair Typing System. Using products aimed toward this hair based of texture and curl pattern, will put you on the road to success in your hair journey. In a later commandment of this book, I will give you great suggestions to incorporate within your hair care product collection. Knowing your hair and the oils suggested has already given you a surface idea as to what you can incorporate into your homemade hair concoctions, or, ingredients you should look for in your hair care products. Now that you are able to classify your hair, you wonder if it is possible to change the pattern of your hair or maybe even the texture of your hair now that you know what you really want right? Next, we will discuss acquiring a different curl pattern.

ACQUIRING A DIFFERENT CURL PATTERN

As a child, my dolls had fair skin, blue or green eyes, blonde hair, with little to no body shape, and because of this, I was not amused. I wanted my dolls to look like me in the beginning, and then I started to prefer them over having darker skin play dolls. My initial reason was not because I wanted to look like them, I was happy with how I looked, but it was because their hair was easier for me to comb and manipulate. The ease of sliding the comb through those blonde strands without tension was bliss compared to a comb through my hair. Of course this, along with mainstream beauty, led me and other little black girls like me, craving straight hair. Getting my hair straightened for special occasions was not enough because I wanted to run my fingers through my hair all the time!

My mother didn't fight with me against my want for straight hair because she was ready to do whatever it took to make it easier for her to manage my hair. Before my curl pattern started to alter, my mother would press my hair straight with a hot comb. What a terrible hair experience! My mother was very careful about this and the hot metal comb rarely ever touched my skin but trust, the sizzle, cracking, and popping of that hot hair grease was enough torture by itself!

 Keeping my hair straight for long periods of time were impossible because any moisture would revert my hair back to its original kinky self. To avoid this from happening, I avoided playing too hard because that would make my roots puffy, and, I would prevent my hair from being in contact with moisture from showering. We created a viscous cycle with hair breakage because I kept my hair dry hair all the time. One day, someone gave my mother the bright idea to give me a kiddie perm to help with the breakage and also, to help make my hair manageable. What better advice was there without much advice or help available? My mother did the best that she could, sometimes I would see growth, sometimes I would see a digression in length; there was always a shuffle of products and techniques being put to the test.

There are a variety of things that you can do to alter the curl pattern of your hair, permanently and temporarily. Your texture will not change much through altering your curl pattern with permanent or temporary processes, but your curl pattern will and can change dramatically.

Permanently altering your curl pattern can be done so in a variety of ways, one option is to relax your hair with a chemical relaxer. This is the appropriate treatment for curly hair. For this treatment, you are straightening your hair with a chemical relaxer application and applying it to your hair preferably with an applicator tool. Perming adds curls to your hair so this is best done on Type 1 hair. When referring to relaxing the hair, some may refer to this process as perming the hair, this is not the appropriate terminology to use but it has become a synonymous term to some. Texturizing your hair, or using a texturizer, is like using a weak strength chemical relaxer treatment. Perming, relaxing, or texturizing your hair permanently alters the curl pattern of your hair. Some hair types are more defiant against chemical treatments than others so some hair types may need multiple treatments to take to the chemicals, or may not. Permanent curl altering treatments are best left to the professionals who went to school to know what is best for your hair. Your typical "kitchen beautician" (home stylists with little to no hair education) can only extend their helping hand so far to help you reach your hair needs.

Temporarily altering your curl pattern does not involve chemical treatments. Using heat or hair rollers will allow your hair to take on the shape of your choice, while simultaneously keeping the very nature of your strands 100% revertible when your hair comes in contact with moisture. When altering your curl pattern with heat, low heat and infrequent use of heat is best to keep your hair revertible. Another manipulating option is to use hair rollers. Using hair rollers to set your hair while wet, will allow it to dry to the shape of your tool and give you the option to sport a different curl with your hair.

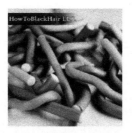

Flexi rods are a popular choice of hair rollers.

In the next COMMANDMENT, we will open up the discussion and the reasons behind using chemical relaxer treatments and also about heat training natural hair.

COMMANDMENT II

THOU SHALT FLEE FROM RELAXERS, TEXTURIZERS, AND HEAT

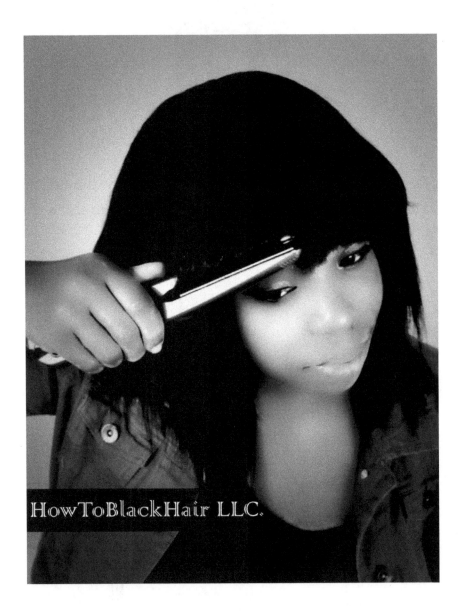

INTRODUCTION TO COMMANDMENT II

OH THE JOYS OF RELAXERS!

Oh the joys of relaxers! A relaxer treatment can produce beautiful results while also leaving you with the worst scalp burns you may ever experience in your life! Sitting in the chair with my hair submerged in relaxer solution, and a towel wrapped around my neck, used to be the life I lived, loved, and hated in the same breath. It was normal no matter whose house I decided to visit, for someone to receive a fresh relaxer treatment from the salon, or a kitchen beautician would grace the presence of a friend of mine, to give the gift of having straight hair once again. From someone with a very sensitive scalp, on top of mild eczema, a relaxer treatment was my devil in disguise! Honestly, it was the biggest temptation for me to touch up the roots of my hair or decide to deal with my hair "au naturel".

At the age of 18, I decided to go natural. It happened with one thought,

> *"I am tired of relaxing my hair and suffering: no more."*

That was all it took for me. I knew very little when it came to hair care even though I was great at styling hair. I suffered going natural because of my lack of knowledge and that is the culprit if you are having a difficult time with maintaining healthy hair. The initial experience when going natural with my hair was that I felt like I was driving to an unknown destination without any directions or guidance. That did not matter to me because I would rather be lost and eventually make it to a destination, than experience that creamy crack ever again!

As you may notice, I hate having relaxer treatments. It became completely unnecessary and when I actually sat back and asked myself a pivotal question, it set me on a new and exciting experience within my hair journey.

WHY DO YOU RELAX YOUR HAIR?

Some things you never really pay attention to unless you actually sit back and question every little thing that you do, or, until someone nonchalantly opens up a thought for you. Let's discuss the reason(s) behind why you are chemically relaxing your hair.

You Have Always Relaxed Your Hair

If this is the reason alone, you may have never actually seen your hair in its natural form. You probably don't think too much of it at all because there are no reasons why you should or should not continue with relaxer treatments. This was my reason for relaxing my hair in addition to having mild eczema, and liking straight hair. If you like your hair how it is and you have no desire to change things, stick with it. But if you only relax your hair because you have always relaxed your hair, why operate as a habitu é ? Maybe you will actually prefer having natural hair over relaxed hair.

Your Hair Is Unmanageable Without It

If this is the reason alone, you have a hard time dealing with your hair when your roots are not relaxed. Having unmanageable hair is not the fault of your hair; it is truly yours because you lack knowledge. The knowledge you know about your hair will transform into a healthy, manageable head of hair. If you do not know what to do to keep your natural hair in a manageable state, it is only natural that you reject the idea of giving up the relaxer. Do not be afraid, if you only relax your hair because it is unmanageable, it is time to learn how to do what works for natural hair and because of that, I am happy that you are reading this book.

You Like Having Straight Hair

If this is the reason alone, you simply love having the look of straight hair! The versatility of hair is endless no matter if your hair is in a processed state, or natural state. This was one of my reasons as to why I had a stronghold to relaxers as well. Also, I loved wearing extensions and my hair was covered all the time with minimum leave out so I asked myself what was the point? I can wear a full sew in with straight hair! But wait what if I want it to look like my hair is actually growing out of my scalp? To get that effect, I would wear Invisible Part Sew In Hairstyles (lace frontals are also a great option). If you only relax your hair to wear straight hairstyles, broaden your horizon to the world of hair extensions while still having natural hair underneath.

You Don't Like Wearing Your Natural Hair

If this is the reason alone, I understand. You probably don't like to see yourself with natural hair while you may also like how natural hair looks on others. There could be some things that you want to unearth so dig a little bit deeper within yourself, to reveal to yourself, why you feel that way. Does natural hair make you feel unfeminine? Why? Is it because your hair will be short? Do you hate how short hair looks on you? Your hair is too loose or tight of curl pattern for your liking? These questions can go on for pages and only you can answer these questions so be honest with yourself. The reason why you do not want to go natural with your hair is attached to a fear that you have within yourself. Stop being afraid and be what you want to be with your hair. Fear is False, Evidence, Appearing, Real! Make baby steps towards fearlessness, it's your hair so rock it how YOU truly want!

You Don't Know How People Will Receive Your Hair

If this is the reason alone, this can be a hard decision making reason for you, because this is a combination of how you think you will receive yourself, and, the fact that you also have no clue as to how others will receive you as well. It is not best for me to tell you to continue to relax your hair, or to go ahead and go natural, because there are many factors you should honestly consider like the opinions of your spouse and job. The reason why I did not say family is because you should be able to count on the fact that they will not disown you because of what naturally grows out of your head. I also did not mention children as a reason because they are usually the most open and unfiltered human beings on this planet. They may insensitively say things because as you know, kids say the darnest things! Children are still growing individuals, not really set in their ways, and usually more open to change if you explain things to them at their level of understanding.

In the workplace, individuality is usually not acceptable. If you were hired for a specific job with your hair displayed natural or with hair extensions, expect to carry on that image to keep your job. Natural hair is still not widely accepted as "professional hair" so if you were hired by your employer with natural hair, that's perfect! If you were hired wearing extensions, please do not retreat from that because you don't know how much you hair had an effect on your opportunity of employment. There have been many situations in which black women and men have lost their jobs for deciding to display the hair that they were naturally born with in the workplace. Of course this is not fair to be judged by what your hair looks like but it happens all the time. Take tattoos for example, for some jobs, like an edgy clothing store, tattoos are probably acceptable. For a news anchor, a visible tattoo would not be acceptable. Remember that your job is not the proper place you should expect to freely display your individuality, there is an image you must hold. If this is a problem for you, don't expect the game to change by your voicing on this matter, look into other places of employment or simply go into business for yourself. Keep in mind that you do not have to sacrifice the health of your hair for your job, wearing weaves or extensions is a great option without having to sacrifice the health of your hair.

On the other hand, your spouse is the person whose opinion weighs heavy, next to yours, because this is the person that you are committing yourself to. You can do with your hair what you want but naturally, you want your spouse to be happy with your decision too. This is the perfect time to talk to your spouse about this topic. Tell him/her what you plan on doing, show pictures and examples of what different types of curl patterns look like and ask them their thoughts about it based on all scenarios. But what if your spouse utterly rejects natural hair? You still have to decide, I can't decide for you. There are a lot of couples who decide to break up because their spouse will not accept them with the hair that naturally grows out of their scalp, while others conform. Based on the seriousness of your relationship, it may be a difficult or easy decision to make in relation to the union between you and that person. Seeing your loved one with hair you have never seen them with before can be a shock but, it usually grows on everyone. Their unease with the hair you were born with should not make you an unacceptable partner to them. Again, you have to make the decision for yourself and whatever decision you choose, let it be the decision you truly want to make for yourself.

HEAT TRAINING YOUR HAIR

Heat training your hair can be detrimental to many, but you can still have success with this hair straightening process. You can also have success with chemically relaxing your hair as well, many do. The focus of this subject is not to teach you how to have success with heat training or relaxing your hair because that would contradict the very nature of this book. So let us understand what heat training is actually doing to your hair.

Heat training your hair decreases the moisture levels and the protein structure of your hair. Using heat tools such as hot combs, blow dryers and flat irons/ smoothing irons dries your hair out on the outside of your hair strands as well as inside of your hair strands. This is the reason why it is difficult for some to heat train their hair without hair damage. The very act of heating your hair with hot tools inflicts damage upon your strands, to some degree, whether you experience unnoticeable (none), minimum, or extreme hair damage/breakage. Remember that ethnic hair is the driest of hair types so providing an even dryer environment may bring you results that you may not want such as: heat trained hair that will not revert while also being damaged as well.

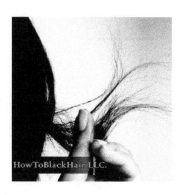

Heat training your hair also weakens the protein structure of your hair; which is what heat trainees want to do to stop their hair from reverting back to its natural curl pattern. Heat training your hair properly, is done with consistent use of heat over time, so that you can avoid excessive hair damage. Any type of hair process promising you bone straight hair, in one session, that is sure to last for weeks/months, is something you want to be cautious of (for example, Brazilian Keratin Blowout Treatments). Frequent use of heat on your hair will naturally begin to break up the protein bonds in your hair. The protein bonds in your hair is responsible for the nature of your hair texture and curl pattern. You will notice a significant difference when heat training your hair, that your curl pattern will appear "weakened" when your hair comes in contact with water.

The same thing that happens at a cellular level inside of your hair strands when heat training your hair, also happens when you relax your hair. When chemically relaxing your hair, you are chemically disturbing the nature of protein bonds in your hair. The chemicals in relaxers are designed to permanently stop the protein bonds in your hair from reconnecting again.

That is what makes this hair process irreversible; you will not continue to have your original curl pattern. The visible hair that you had relaxer applied to will be permanently straightened. Chemical relaxers are also thought to be linked to breast cancer and thyroid issues. There are many personal testimonies that believe this to be the case even though there is no scientific evidence, to date, to support this claim at this time. These claims have been made by many stylists who have given chemical relaxer treatments, and by those who have been on the receiving end of a relaxer treatment as well. This piece of information is not said to purposefully deter you from chemically relaxing your hair, it is said to give you an idea as to the possible effects that a relaxer treatment may have on your health.

Both of these acts, heat training and relaxing your hair, are irreversible on your visible hair strands and in some cases, relaxing your hair can permanently destroy your hair follicles and cause alopecia. If you want to once again embrace the way your hair naturally takes form when grown out of your scalp, you have to cut off the "trained hair" because it will not revert back to what your hair naturally is. There is nothing you can do to reconnect those protein cells you have purposefully broken through heat training and relaxer treatments. You have to cut that hair if you no longer want that look for your hair.

Heat training is not a suggested option for those who are choosing to finally go natural because it can become a crutch for new naturals when adjusting to their natural hair. The infamous Catch-22 that plays out is the common situation of having natural hair while wearing straight extension partial sews ins, and using heat to blend your leave out with your extensions. The Catch-22 of this act is that neither options are desirable but one option has to be made if you decide to place yourself in this situation. You will either have leave out that is not properly blended or a heat trained leave out that will not revert back to your natural pattern.

To summarize this commandment, if thou canst go natural without forsaking heat tools, thou must consider what makes relaxer treatments any more different?

In the next commandment, COMMANDMENT III, we will discuss the topic of cutting your damaged ends.

COMMANDMENT III

THOU MUST CUT YOUR DAMAGED ENDS

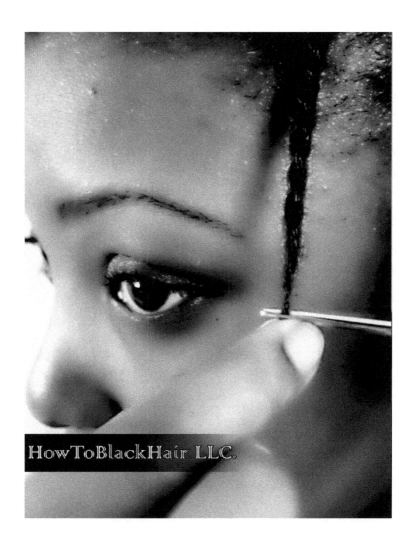

HowToBlackHair LLC.

INTRODUCTION TO COMMANDMENT III

DECIDING TO GO NATURAL

Deciding to go natural was an easy decision for me to make because I was so ready to give up chemically relaxing my hair. I was willing to do whatever it took to have a healthy, thick, full head of hair without having to rely on a relaxer. Right after coming back from my Honeymoon in the Bahamas, I threw away every hair product that revolved around relaxed hair. The first thing I chucked towards the trash can was my half-filled containers of kiddie relaxers that I had in my freezer, along with other hair products. I have no real reason as to why I used to keep my leftover store bought relaxer kits in the freezer; someone must have told me that it keeps the solution fresh and effective when you want to touch up your roots.

So, as you may have guessed, just about every hair product I owned was gone. The only items that I had left were a wide tooth comb, shampoo, conditioner and moisturizing hair lotion. The next thing that I did was research, research, research. I wanted to know exactly what I needed to do to take care of my natural hair and in the meantime, I infamously wore Box Braids, wigs, and Full Sew In Hairstyles. Every bit of information I came across when trying to develop a regimen always told me to combat hair damage by cutting of damaged ends. Damaged ends included natural damage like split ends and single strand knots, along with, relaxed, texturized, and heat trained ends. Every time I would read information on cutting off my ends, I automatically rejected the validity of their knowledge about hair and began to take everything with a grain of salt. Because of my stubbornness, I became idle in my hair journey. I finally began to accept the information that I wanted to, while at the same time, always overlooking reasons why trimming/cutting your hair is important for having healthy hair.

Looking back on this situation makes me laugh at myself, because in my mind, I thought I knew what was necessary and what was not when clearly I had no idea. Slowly but surely, my relaxed ends began to break off and my hair began to look thicker and less sparse. This gave me the false conclusion that my hair did not need a trim because it was "taking care of itself". As time went on, I noticed that the ends of my hair started to thin and feel dry, and since the oldest part of your hair are the ends of your hair, I assumed that it was time to start deep conditioning more often, even though I was deep conditioning once a week. My roots felt wonderful but my ends were so troublesome when I tried to wear twist outs or an afro.

As much as I tried to hang on to my wispy straw-like ends, I finally came to the conclusion that it was time for the big chop.

Big Chop: the process of cutting relaxed or permed ends of one's hair when transitioning from chemically processed hair to natural hair.

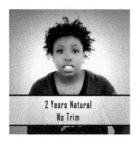
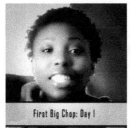
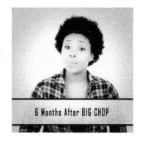

2 Years Natural
No Trim

First Big Chop: Day 1

6 Months After BIG CHOP

What a huge difference it was to cut off my damaged hair, I could not believe it! Looking back, I felt like a picture that I had seen of the back of a black woman's head, who was riding on a city bus. Her hair was barely long enough to squeeze into a ponytail, with about an inch of damaged relaxed hair at the ends of her roots, and the picture captioned, "I want to go natural but I'm so scared." Looking back, I can now make light of that situation and laugh about it but I know exactly how she, along with others, feel during that phase. I was not afraid to have natural hair; I just did not want to have short hair. I used to feel like long hair was the only beautiful hair and that is why so many women suffer with extremely damaged hair, just for the sake of keeping as much length as possible. I refused to cut my hair when in reality, if I would have sooner, it would have been about 4 times longer than the "6 months after BIG CHOP" photo above. As soon as I cut the ends of my hair, it started to blossom like a beautiful flower. If you still have not cut off your damaged ends, you are purposefully dragging your feet on your hair journey. Next, we will talk about if dry hair actually means damaged hair because it can be confusing trying to understand the difference.

DOES DRY HAIR MEAN DAMAGE

Determining the appropriate circumstance for cutting your damaged or unwanted ends is difficult to do if you don't know what to look for. When cutting your hair, you only want to cut off what is necessary and nothing more. It is a common mistake for someone to cut off too much unwanted hair and I will help you to understand what is necessary so that you can make sure this does not happen to you. Also, in most cases, it is best to place your confidence in a stylist who specializes in cutting hair. So before we begin to understand how to cut off unwanted hair effectively, let us first understand what dry hair means. Note that dry hair can take on a variety of forms and appear to be damage when in fact, your hair simply lacks moisture.

Dry Hair: hair that lacks the necessary moisture to retain a soft, smooth appearance.

When caring for your hair, this will be an inevitable hair experience from time to time. Your hair can become dry because of constant manipulation and even your diet. Also, regularly wetting your hair, the quality of your tools, and also the quality of your hair products has an enormous impact on the health of your hair as well. Since there is much information to share on the health of your hair in terms of your frequent use of water, the quality of your tools and the quality of your hair products, these things will be discussed, in detail, in the next commandment. To begin, we will focus on how constant manipulation can be a direct link to hair damage.

CONSTANT MANUPULATION

Constant manipulation will cause your hair to become dry no matter how well you take care of your hair. You could be using the best daily moisturizing cream to have ever graced this Earth but again, constant manipulation can and will dry your hair out.

Another reason why constant manipulation is a problem is because your skin will absorb water from your hair. Maybe you have not thought much about it, but human skin is pretty absorbent! Did you know that during a 5 minute shower, your skin can absorb about a quarter of a gallon of water? This is why your skin swells and your finger pads wrinkle after a long bath: it has actually absorbed water. Skin is water resistant, not water proof, so constantly stroking and touching your hair can draw moisture away from your strands. It is best to only touch your hair when it is necessary such as styling or rearranging your style unto your liking. Casually twirling your fingers around your ringlets or fidgeting your fingers through your hair, on a constant basis, is a sure way to deplete moisture from your hair overtime. Also your frequency of styling is best left up to your preference. There is no rule that says styling your hair x amount of times is wrong, just keep in mind that the longer you can maintain a style without manipulation, the more opportunity you provide for healthy thriving hair. In addition to your skin absorption being a reason for experiencing dry hair, constant manipulation also strips the outer protective barriers that keep water sealed within your hair.

Constantly manipulating your hair strips away your natural produced oil (sebum) and it also weakens the scales that form a protective barrier around the strands of your hair. Everyone naturally secretes sebum all over their body with our scalp being the place where the most sebum is produced. Those who have more kinky and curly textures generally produce slightly less sebum than others who have different hair types and curl patterns; so naturally, having a dry scalp is also an issue along with having naturally drier hair. Combing or brushing your hair may seem like the thing to do to help sebum distribute throughout your hair but this will only do more bad than good if this amount of manipulation is more than what is necessary to produce a style.

Now let us talk about the scales on the outside of your hair strands, these scales can be seen under a microscope but not to the naked eye. To understand the physicality of your hair scales, grab a section of your own hair and hold it out as taut (stretched) as possible. Now take the fingers of your free hand and rub your hair downward starting at the roots toward the ends of your hair. This can be done on wet or dry hair and it should feel very smooth. Now carefully rub your fingers from the bottom of your section of hair sliding your way up to your roots. You will feel much resistance! Your scales naturally lay on the outside of your hair strands, fashioned in a downward motion, to keep in water and nutrients, and to also block out the elements. Constantly manipulating your hair will naturally weaken your hair scales which leave the innermost part of your strands exposed. This allows more water and nutrients to be lost through evaporation thus, leaving you with dry hair.

DIET

Your diet is important to the health of your body, and also to the health of your hair. As your body goes through hormonal changes triggered by age, pregnancy, puberty and even medicine, you can usually point to one of those reasons as to what is causing undesirable effects on your hair. Those independent reasons can affect the quality of your health and hair but for this specific discussion, we will focus on the effects that diet alone has on the quality of your hair.

There are times when our cravings will make it hard to resist those temptations that we try to ignore and from time to time, it is ok to give in, it is natural to crave the things that you enjoy. An occasional slice of cheesecake or take out from an oriental restaurant will not dry your hair to smithereens, let's be realistic! What matters is how often we consume things that are not so good for use because the quality of our diet is very important and reflective in the health of your hair. Eating a diet high in processed foods is sure to make you an unhealthy person! Foods high in saturated fats, sugars, and salts, leave little to no room for your daily intake of nutrients. Food consumed closer to its natural state, will be a better option for you for the sake of your health and hair. Instead of potato chips, eat dehydrated kale chips and instead or ice cream, try frozen yogurt.

At the end of the day, if you have not consumed enough vitamins and minerals through your food and drinks, there will not be enough supply to go around so your extremities will suffer. Our body does a great job showing that we are lacking certain vitamins and nutrients, for example; thinning hair, brittle nails, sensitive teeth, and even hair loss are a few warning signs. Just think, if you do not drink much water, or at least aim to drink the daily amount suggested, how much water will be left for your hair after your vital organs receive their share? The beauty of our body is that it prioritizes what is consumed to keep us healthy and alive, first and foremost. You hair, nails, and skin comes in last place to receive water and nutrients in comparison to your brain, heart, and other vital organs. The moral of a quality diet (eating habits) is that you want to focus on being internally healthy more than your focus may be on finding the product that fixes a persistent problem.

To summarize this commandment, we have explored two important reasons that differentiate hair damage from dry hair. A simple question you can ask yourself to know the difference between the two is,

"Is the condition of my hair reversible or irreversible?"

Dry hair becomes reversible as soon as you come to the conclusion of what is causing your hair to be dry. Hair damage is irreversible because there is nothing you can do to change the condition of your hair such as; split ends, single strand knots, heat damage, and permanent curl/texture alternating treatments.

In the next commandment, COMMANDMENT IV, we will explore how important water is to the quality of your hair.

COMMANDMENT IV

WATER; NO OTHER PRODUCT SHALL COME BEFORE ME

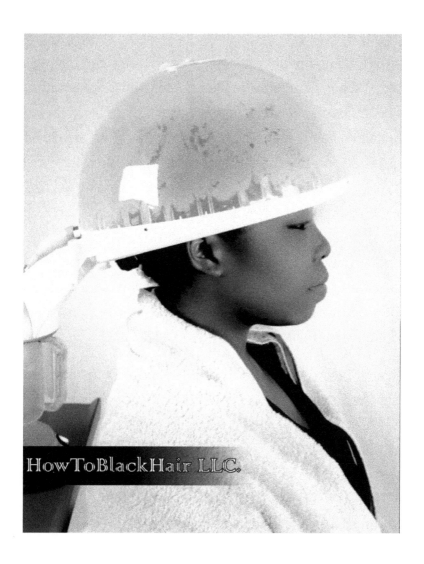

INTRODUCTION TO COMMANDMENT IV

THE RELATIONSHIP MY HAIR AND WATER HAD

The relationship my hair and water had, during the time when I had relaxed hair, was pretty much nonexistent. Water only touched my hair to remove any hair products or build up I had on my hair. When it was time to clean my hair, water was used to rinse shampoo from my strands. When I dyed my hair with box dye, or chemically relaxed my hair, water was used to remove those products. Never did I view water as a necessary source of moisture because I did not think to moisturize my hair with water but with oils and moisture promising hair products. Keeping water away from my hair, until it was time to rid my hair of product or buildup, was an unwritten rule many relaxed girls I knew lived by.

I remember being a pre-teen in middle school choosing my hair over my grade in PE class. I knew that it was going to be a problem for me to pass my PE class because it involved two things that I was not too fond of, in relation to my hair, was sweating and swimming. The latest time that I could postpone my PE credit was in the 7th grade and sadly, that is exactly what I did. When it was finally time to take my PE class, I suffered a horrible participation score in gym and swim. Attendance was a third of my grade and participation made up the majority so even though I had perfect attendance, I always tinkered between having a D or F letter grade. If I did not have this required credit for physical education, I could not graduate middle school.

Often I would appear to "feel sick" in class, which only worked for a little while being that my grade weighed heavily on participation. It literally depressed me knowing that I was allowing my hair to control my academics. I always did just enough in gym class and swim class to show that I was trying when in reality, I was not. I, along with other relaxed girls, sat out on the sideline when it was time to swim and of course, everyone blamed Mother Nature.

The point of chemically relaxing your hair is to stop your natural curl pattern from reverting when it is in contact with moisture (water). There should be no fear of water being in contact with your hair at that point in all honesty. Yes your hair and/or roots may become a little puffy but with care, you can keep your hair tame. Your hair should never get in the way of your life. You shall never be ruled by your hair: that is unacceptable.

This hair commandment will ease your hair care worries when it comes to swimming with your natural hair. I will walk you through a step by step process that applies simultaneously to swimming in both chlorinated water and salt water. Also, this commandment will go into detail on refreshing (hydrating) your curls during times when you hair starts to feel dry, even though it is not quite time to shampoo wash your hair. Refreshing (hydrating) your hair can be done without having to experience a wash session. The world of co-washing and spritzing your hair will be explained later in this commandment

SWIMMING WITH NATURAL HAIR

Swimming with natural hair can be a detrimental or wonderful experience, depending on how well you are prepared for the occasion. Being afraid to get your hair wet because it may ruin the desired condition you want your hair to be in, needs to be a thing of the past. To swim with natural hair, we will go step by step, in detail, on what you want to do before and after swimming, without risking the health of your hair. The detailed steps you must follow when swimming with natural hair applies to the same conditions if you arc wcaring a weave, extensions or natural hair styles.

Before Swimming

1. Your Hair Must Be Stretched

This is the most important part of your preparation because free hair, hair that is not contained in either braids or twists, will tangle. This creates the ultimate environment for single strand knots to thrive, especially if your hair is coily.

Single Strand Knot (Fair Knot): the process of a hair strand coiling upon itself and creating a miniature knot on the end of itself; hence a single strand knot. Unraveling them by hand will squander your time, cutting the knots is best.

 If you are wearing weaves or extensions, you still want your hair to be in twists or braids.

For example, these are some hairstyles that would be fitting for swimming; Box Braids, Micro Braids, Cornrow Braids, Senegalese Twists, Kinky Twists, Mini Twists and Two Strand Twists, just to name a few.

A hair style that would not be fitting would be a; Twist Out, Braid Out, Mini Twist Out, Flat Twist Out, and especially an Afro

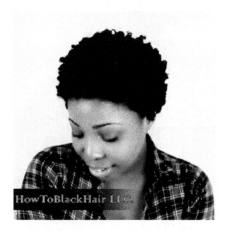

Picture of A Bantu Knot Out

2. Saturate Your Hair With Water

Thoroughly saturate your hair with tap water, shower water, or filtered water, whichever you are used to using for your hair.

Rinsing your hair with filtered water is the better choice but, if you do not rinse or wash your hair with filtered water, you do not have to go out of your way to do so for swimming.

Also, the reason why this step is necessary, even though your hair is going to be in chlorine water, is because allowing your hair to absorb chlorine water can be damaging to your hair. Chlorine molecules weigh down your hair and this can cause hair breakage/hair damage. Swimming in either chlorine water or salt water, with already wet hair, makes it difficult for your hair to absorb chlorine water and/or salt water.

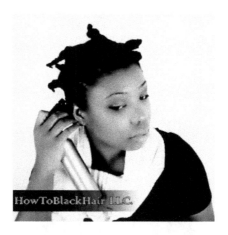

In this step, it is also a good idea to wear a good quality swimmers cap that will not allow water in. If you have such a cap, you do not have to saturate your hair before swimming. It is optional if you still want to wet your hair before swimming and wear a swimming cap to cover your wet hair, but it is not necessary.

After Swimming

1. Shampoo Wash Your Hair

After you have finished swimming it is now time to shampoo your hair. If you have to take care of immediate responsibilities like tending to children for example, or going to another location that does not allow you the chance to wash your hair, immediately rinse your hair with water and shampoo your hair when you get the chance.

This is why it is important to thoroughly saturate your hair with water first, before going swimming in either chlorine water or salt water, to better care for your hair after swimming.

If you did not choose to saturate your hair with water before going swimming, you have to use a chelating (key-lay-ting) shampoo to immediately wash your hair after swimming, a quick water rinse is not best in this situation. Chelating shampoos are specially formulated to remove chlorine from your hair and in this case, you have to use a chelating shampoo to wash your hair after swimming.

If your hair was saturated with water before swimming, shampooing your hair with a chelating shampoo is not necessary for preserving the health of your hair; using a chelating shampoo or your regular shampoo to wash your hair, in this case, does not matter.

2. Deep Condition Your Hair

If before swimming, your hair was in its ideal condition, you do not have to deep condition your hair, this step is optional.

Deep conditioning your hair is mandatory if you were experiencing hair problems out of its ideal condition before or after swimming. If you are currently experiencing problems with your hair being constantly dry, it is best to deep condition your hair after you shampoo wash your hair. You can choose to deep condition without a plastic cap, with a plastic cap and/or a towel wrapped around your cap, or under a warm hooded dryer. The deep conditioning methods, in previous order, will meet the need for mildly dry hair, intermediately dry hair, and chronically dry hair. Choose which deep conditioning process best applies to you, according to your situation and circumstance.

3. Seal In Moisture With Oil

Sealing in moisture: applying a coating of oil on wet or damp hair to slow down the rate of water evaporation from your hair.

Applying oil onto your hair while it is damp or wet, does not PERMANATELY stop water from evaporating from your hair. Sealing in your moisture with oil keeps your hair moisturized for a longer period of time, when in comparison to hair that has fully dried before any oil was applied.

The key to sealing in moisture well is to do so on hair that is not dripping wet. Also, make sure to apply just enough oil onto your hair that does not leave your hair feeling oily. That is why it is important to understand the physicality of your hair by using the LOIS Hair Typing System and the Andre Walker Hair Typing System (Commandment I). Use both hair typing systems to determine which oils would be best to seal water into your strands, and of course, not all hair is typical, so experiment to see which oil(s) work best for your hair.

This is the last hair care step you need to implement after going swimming. You have braided, twisted or banded your hair, saturated your hair in water, swam, rinsed or shampooed, deep conditioned (optional), and sealed in moisture with oil to prevent dry hair.

Based on your hair needs and what feels best with your hair, you may wish to apply oil onto your hair as soon as it stops dripping. In most cases, the prime opportunity to apply oil onto hair is hair that is about 10% to 30% dry. This prevents you from applying too much oil onto your hair and also, prevents the chance of water drip from your hair again, due to the added weight of oil on your hair.

These tips are golden fail-proof keys for healthy hair care when swimming. You never have to complicate natural hair, the more simple your techniques are, the more control you have over the state of your hair. With only four hair care steps to implement when swimming, along with one optional step, you never have to worry about swimming again with your natural hair.

Now that you know how to swim with natural hair, let us understand what is means to refresh (hydrate) our hair and when it is necessary.

REFRESHING YOUR CURLS

You will be introduced to the world of refreshing (hydrating) your hair by co-washing or spritzing your hair. We will first focus on co-washing your hair for moisture and then on spritzing your hair for moisture.

CO-WASHING

Co-Wash: conditioner washing your hair to restore moisture into your hair to combat dryness.

Conditioner washing your hair does not replace cleaning your hair with cleansing agents (shampoo). The purpose of conditioner washing your hair is to provide maximum moisture that you need to combat dry hair, when it is not necessary for you to shampoo wash your hair. You may be one of many who have the freedom to shampoo infrequently, if you do not have much natural buildup, or product buildup, on your hair and scalp.

Also you will simultaneously perform the act of co-washing your hair for the detangling process, which will be discussed in a later commandment.

SPRITZING

Spritzing: lightly misting your hair when a co -wash is not necessary but, you still need moisture.

The need to spritz your hair, in most cases, is best for hair that is bound in styles like twists and braids. Spritzing your hair daily is the best technique you want to implement when reaching your hair through extensions and weaves. Spritz your hair if you need light moisture to keep your hair supple and moisturized. If you need to wet your hair past the point of generally misting your hair, the better choice is to co-wash for great moisture.

To summarize this commandment, you now understand that water is not the enemy, in fact, water is the best product for your hair! In the beginning of this commandment, we discussed how important water is in the preparation of swimming with natural hair. Water is a barrier of protection for your hair against chlorine water and salt water. Water also restores moisture that you need to hydrate your hair by conditioner washing your hair or, by spritzing your hair with water. Healthy natural hair thrives when water (moisture) is present and in addition to keeping your hair moisturized, good hair care techniques (along with the right products) aligns you on the path to having great healthy thriving natural hair.

In the next commandment, COMMANDMENT V, we will discuss that very thing; implementing a healthy hair care regimen along with using the right products to achieve your best hair.

COMMANDMENT V

THOU SHALL AIM TO USE NATURAL HAIR PRODUCTS

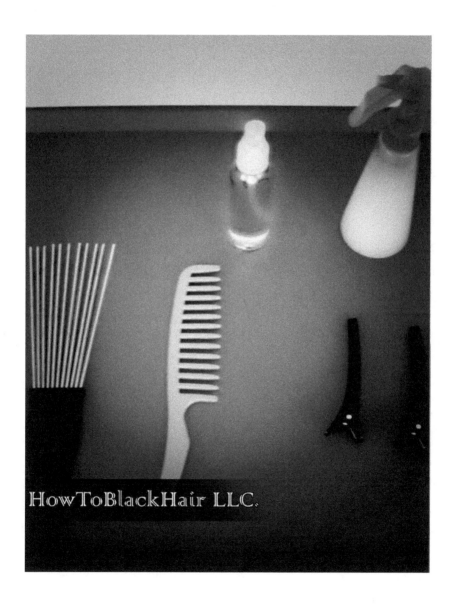

HowToBlackHair LLC.

INTRODUCTION TO COMMANDMENT V

THE BEAUTY SUPPLY STORE WAS MY SAFE HAVEN

The beauty supply store was my safe haven: always there for me in time of my needs and wants. I remember being a young girl bursting with excitement every Friday or Saturday to buy new barrettes, hair knockers, or my favorite, braiding hair. Buying braiding hair meant that I might have a little braid design on the side (depending on the braider) or I might have medium sized cornrow extensions. This was a short lived moment that gave me the chance to finally have long hair once again. At this age, I had no idea about weaves yet, I always thought the women my mother's age had really good perms or at least had "good hair".

As I got older and finally settled into my teenage years, I was already weaving, braiding, and relaxing my own hair and the hair store felt different this time around. I no longer burst with excitement; I needed to buy my "hair fix". I was never without a weave or some type of extension. Being that I was still a minor, no one would hire me so I did not have a job to buy my hair products. The money I had to buy my hair products was money that I would make from braiding hair in high school. I braided my friend's hair, their friend's hair; everyone who had hair and liked braids eventually paid me to braid their hair from school too!

I felt invincible in the hair store when I needed to purchase new hair. If I wanted a long straight look, I would buy 10 to 14 inches of weave (wefted hair) in a kinky Yaki Texture. Having wispy layers staggering down my back was my favorite look being that it looked most realistic for my hair. A pass of the flat straightening iron on this hair texture blended effortlessly with my relaxed hair. When my friends want a weave or extension (non wefted hair) I knew exactly how to pick their right texture whether they had Silky Yaki or Regular Yaki textured hair. Sadly, I had no idea how to choose the right hair care products to maintain what was underneath my weaves and extensions.

It was difficult trying to figure out the right tools I needed because I did not know how to decipher through the ingredients located on the back of the label. I used the title and description located on the front of hair products to lead me to my decision. If the bottle lacked style and creativity, what was inside the bottle, probably had what I did not want. If the contents smelled fragrant, the product was considered. So at checkout, I had the prettiest, most colorful and most fragrant hair creams and hair products to purchase. Of course I was disappointed every single time. This was one of many situations that frustrated me to the point of figuring out what ingredients I needed in my products to take care of my hair. I was tired of disappointing myself and I was definitely tired of wasting my money.

I had come to the conclusion that hair becomes difficult when your hair practices and products become more difficult and harder to understand. My hair products had ingredients in it that I first off, could not pronounce and other ingredients seemed just unnecessary. Why do I need Red 40 color and Lake Blue color in my shampoo? Does this provide anything of value to my hair, I don't think so! The best hair products seem to have simple basic ingredients that were easy to pronounce, while meeting your hair needs.

In this commandment, we will explore the ingredients that you want and do not want in your hair products before you decide to purchase them. Also, natural homemade products will be suggested in this commandment to provide exactly what you will need in your hair care regimen as an alternative to store bought products. In the next commandment, a walkthrough of your hair care process will be explored as well to help assist you further when caring for your natural hair. Knowing the best hair care products to use will provide the opportunity to wear weaves and extensions as an accessory, and not as a mask for unhealthy damaged hair.

INGREDIENTS IN YOUR HAIR CARE PRODUCTS

The ingredients that you use in your hair care products affect the quality of your hair. Even though your hair care techniques are just as important as your hair products, using non purposed hair ingredients in your hair products is the culprit, in many cases, for unruly hair that has become hard to manage. We will explore the products that you want and do not want to have in your hair care ingredients.

SHAMPOO

SAFE INGREDIENTS	HARSH INGREDIENTS
Water	Ammonium Lauryl Sulfate
Pure Glycerin Soap	Ammonium Laureth Sulfate
Cocomidopropyl Betaine	Sodium Lauryl Sulfate
Cocamindapropyl	Sodium Laureth Sulfate
Hydroxysultaine	Triethanolamine Lauryl
Lauramide Oxide	Sulfate
Lauramide Diethanolamine	Sulfonates
Cocamide Diethanolamine	Disodium Mono Oleamide
(DEA)	Sulfosuccinates
Cocamide	
Monoethanolamine (MEA)	

RINSE CONDITIONER/ DEEP CONDITIONER/
DETANGLING CONDITIONER

SAFE INGREDIENTS	HARSH INGREDIENTS
Water	Petroleum
Olive Oil	Petrolatum
Coconut Oil	Lanolin
Jojoba Oil	Bee's Wax
Avocado Oil	Dimethicone
Peanut Oil	Dimethiconol
Mango Oil/Butter	Behenoxy Dimethicone
Almond Oil/Butter	Phenyl Trimethicone
Shea Oil/Butter	Simethicone
Grapeseed Oil	Trimethicone
Cocoa Butter	Polydimethysiloxane
Tea Tree Oil	Cyclomethicone
Peppermint Oil	Cyclopentasiloxane
Castor Oil	Trimethylsiloxysilicates
Honey	PEG Modified Dimethicone
Glycerin	Dimethicone Copolyol
Glycerides	
Pathenol	
Cellulose	
Polyquarternium -10	
Polyquarternium -7	
Lauric Acid (Lauryl Acid)	
Stearic Acid (Stearyl Acid)	
Oleic Acid (Oleyl Acid)	
Linoleic Acid	
Cetyl Acid	
Behenyl Acid	
Cetyl Alchohol	

MOISTURIZERS (conditioner ingredient list applies)

STYLING GELS/POMADES

SAFE INGREDIENTS	HARSH INGREDIENTS
Water Carbomer Hydrolyzed Wheat Protein Aloe Vera Gel/Juice	Alcohol REFER TO HARSH INGREDIENTS ON ALL LISTS

STYLING TOOLS

SAFE TOOLS	HARSH TOOLS
Seamless Wide Tooth Combs Soft Boar Bristle Hair Brush Bobby Pins with balled ends Silk Accessories Seamless Hair Bands Hair Cutting Shears	Combs with seams Plastic Bristle Hair Brush Bobby Pins without balled ends Cotton Accessories Metal/plastic binding Hair Bands Rubber Bands Safety Scissors/Multi Use Scissors

HOMEMADE HAIR CARE PRODUCT RECIPES

You can use the previous categorized lists as a guide for purchasing your staple hair care products. Some hair products that you choose to buy may have new ingredients listed on them, along with other abbreviations that you may not understand. With new chemicals being constructed around the world daily, it becomes difficult trying to figure out if new strains of fatty acids or silicones are safe for use on your hair because in some cases, they may be deemed safe for use before extensive research has been done on that specific ingredient.

A great way to guarantee that you will always have a quality hair product on hand is to make your products yourself of course! There are many hair companies that do a great job of only using natural, quality ingredients in their hair care products. On the other side of the spectrum, some hair companies proclaim that their products are very moisturizing, while their ingredient list contains every form of petrolatum there is! Your quest for finding quality hair care products begins here, provided with lists portrayed earlier in the commandment, to help you. Or, you can choose to create your own hair care products in the comfort of your home.

In order, product recipes and instructions will follow your basic hair care and styling products such as your; Shampoo, Deep Conditioner, Detangling Conditioner, Moisturizer, and a Styling Gel/Pomade. Also, keep in mind that your homemade products are usually free of preservatives so storing your products in a cool, dark place is best for the life of your products.

SHAMPOO

CHAMOMILE SHAMPOO	DIRECTIONS
• 4 Bags Chamomile Tea • 4 TBSP. Pure Soap Flakes • 1 TBSP. Glycerin • 1 ½ CUPS Hot Water • 1 Applicator Bottle • Small mixing bowl • Utensil to stir contents	• Steep tea bags in 1 ½ cups of hot water for 10 minutes. • Remove tea bags, add soap flakes (allow soap to soften). • Mix in glycerin well. • Thoroughly mix all ingredients in the mixing bowl. • Transfer contents into the applicator bottle. • Store any remaining shampoo in a cool, dark place.

AFRICAN BLACK SOAP	DIRECTIONS
<ul><li>4 TBSP. African Black Soap (crumbled)</li><li>1 CUP Hot Water</li><li>4 TBSP. Pure Soap Flakes</li><li>2 TSP. Pure Honey</li><li>3 TSP. Grapeseed Oil</li><li>Container with lid</li><li>Small mixing bowl</li><li>Utensil to stir contents</li></ul>	<ul><li>Thoroughly mix all ingredients in the mixing bowl.</li><li>Transfer contents into the container.</li><li>Store any remaining shampoo in a cool, dark place.</li></ul>

SHAMPOO (Continued)

COCONUT MILK SHAMPOO	DIRECTIONS
<ul><li>¼ CUP Liquid Castile Soap</li><li>3 TBSP. Organic Coconut Milk</li><li>1 TSP. Water</li><li>1 TSP. Safflower Oil</li><li>1 Applicator Bottle</li></ul>	<ul><li>Thoroughly shake contents inside the applicator bottle.</li><li>Store any remaining shampoo in a cool, dark place.</li></ul>

DEEP CONDITIONER

BANANA HONEY DEEP CONDITIONER	DIRECTIONS
<ul><li>1 Large Overripe Banana</li><li>3 TBSP. Extra Virgin Olive Oil</li><li>3 TBSP. Pure Vegetable Glycerin</li><li>2 TBSP. Pure Honey</li><li>Small mixing bowl</li><li>Container with lid</li><li>Hand Blender</li></ul>	<ul><li>Thoroughly blend all contents in your mixing bowl.</li><li>Leave applied all over hair for 30-45 minutes.</li><li>Thoroughly rinse out conditioner with warm water.</li><li>Final rinse with coolest water, you can stand, to close cuticles.</li><li>Store any remaining conditioner in a cool, dark place.</li></ul>

DEEP CONDITIONER (Continued)

COCONUT HONEY DEEP CONDITIONER	DIRECTIONS
• 4 TBSP. Extra Virgin Coconut Oil • 2 TBSP. Pure Honey • 1 Applicator Bottle • Large bowl of hot steaming water	• Add contents into the applicator bottle. • Stand applicator bottle in bowl of hot water until mixture becomes warm. • Thoroughly shake contents inside the applicator bottle. • Leave applied all over hair for 30-45 minutes • Thoroughly rinse with warm water. • Final rinse with coolest water, you can stand, to close cuticles. • Store any remaining conditioner in a cool, dark place.

ADVOCADO DEEP CONDITIONER	DIRECTIONS
• ½ Overripe Avocado • ½ TSP. Coconut Oil • 3 drops of Lavender or Rosemary Essential oil • 1 Applicator Bottle • Small mixing bowl • Utensil to stir/mash contents	• Thoroughly mash/stir ingredients in the mixing bowl. • Add to hair, working from the ends to roots, until you run out of mixture. • Do not worry about coating all of your hair, your ends will benefit the most and requires more conditioner. • Leave applied for 15-20 minutes. • Thoroughly rinse with warm water. • Final rinse with coolest water, you can stand, to close cuticles. • Store any remaining conditioner in a cool, dark place

DETANGLING CONDITIONER

ADVOCADO & VINEGAR DETANGLING CONDITIONER	DIRECTIONS
<ul><li>1 Overripe Avocado</li><li>¼ CUP Extra Virgin Olive Oil</li><li>½ CUP Unrefined Shea Butter</li><li>3 TBSP. Apple Cider Vinegar</li><li>Small mixing bowl</li><li>Container with lid</li><li>Hand Blender</li></ul>	<ul><li>Thoroughly blend all contents in your mixing bowl.</li><li>Saturate your hair, allow to sit for 5 minutes, detangle.</li><li>Thoroughly rinse with warm water.</li><li>Final rinse with coolest water, you can stand, to close cuticles.</li><li>Store any remaining conditioner in a cool, dark place.</li></ul>

SOUR CREAM CUCUMBER DETANGLING CONDITIONER	DIRECTIONS
<ul><li>½ Cucumber</li><li>½ Overripe Avocado</li><li>1/3 CUP Sour Cream</li><li>2 square cubes of any Eggplant (no skin)</li><li>Small mixing bowl</li><li>Container with lid</li><li>Hand Blender</li></ul>	<ul><li>Thoroughly blend all contents in your mixing bowl.</li><li>Saturate your hair, allow to sit for 5 minutes, detangle.</li><li>Thoroughly rinse with warm water.</li><li>Final rinse with coolest water, you can stand, to close cuticles.</li><li>Store any remaining conditioner in a cool, dark place.</li></ul>

GREEK YOGURT DETANGLING CONDITIONER	DIRECTIONS
<ul><li>1 CUP of Greek Yogurt</li><li>2 TBSP. Pure Honey</li><li>6 TBSP. Olive Oil</li><li>1 TSP. Pure Vitamin E Oil</li><li>1 Applicator Bottle</li><li>Small mixing bowl</li><li>Whisk Utensil</li></ul>	<ul><li>Thoroughly whisk all contents in your mixing bowl.</li><li>Transfer contents into the applicator bottle (if fitting).</li><li>Saturate your hair, allow to sit for 5 minutes, detangle.</li><li>Thoroughly rinse with warm water.</li><li>Final rinse with coolest water, you can stand, to close cuticles.</li><li>Store any remaining conditioner in a cool, dark place.</li></ul>

MOISTURIZER

ALOE VERA JUICE CURL REFRESHER	DIRECTIONS
<ul><li>7oz Aloe Vera Juice</li><li>1TBSP. Jojoba Oil</li><li>1TBSP. Avocado Oil</li><li>3 drops of Rosemary Essential Oil</li><li>8 oz. spray bottle</li></ul>	<ul><li>Vigorously shake contents before use.</li><li>Spritz hair to restore needed moisture.</li><li>Store any remaining moisturizer in a cool, dark place.</li></ul>

LANOLIN CREAM MOISTURIZING BUTTER	DIRECTIONS
<ul><li>1oz Lanolin Oil</li><li>1 oz Unrefined Shea Butter</li><li>2 TSP. Extra Virgin Olive Oil</li><li>5 drops of Rosemary Essential Oil</li><li>1TSP. Jojoba Oil</li><li>8 oz. container with lid</li><li>Small mixing bowl</li><li>Hand Blender</li></ul>	<ul><li>Thoroughly blend all contents in your mixing bowl.</li><li>Transfer mixture into the container.</li><li>Store any remaining moisturizer in a cool, dark place.</li></ul>

SHEA BUTTER ALOE MOISTURIZING BUTTER	DIRECTIONS
<ul><li>½ CUP Unrefined Shea Butter</li><li>¼ CUP Aloe Vera Gel</li><li>2 TBSP. Grapeseed Oil</li><li>1 TSP. Pure Honey</li><li>8 oz. container with lid</li><li>Small mixing bowl</li><li>Hand Blender</li></ul>	<ul><li>Thoroughly blend all contents in your mixing bowl.</li><li>Transfer mixture into the container.</li><li>Store any remaining moisturizer in a cool, dark place.</li></ul>

HAIR GEL/POMADE

HONEY FLAXSEED GEL	DIRECTIONS
<ul><li>2 CUPS Water</li><li>¼ CUP Flax Seeds</li><li>1 TBSP. Pure Honey</li><li>½ TSP. Vitamin E Oil</li><li>5 drops of Rosemary Oil</li><li>Container with lid</li><li>Utensil to mash contents</li><li>A sieve (small flower sifter)</li><li>Boiling pot</li></ul>	<ul><li>Boil water and flaxseeds in your pot and stir until jelly like.</li><li>Pour mixture into the sieve and mash with your utensil over your container.</li><li>Thoroughly mix in the rest of your ingredients.</li><li>Allow to set in cool place.</li><li>Store any remaining gel in a cool, dark place.</li></ul>

HAIR GEL/POMADE (Continued)

EGG WHITE HAIR GEL	DIRECTIONS
• 3 Egg Whites • 2/3 CUP Aloe Vera Gel • 2 TBSP. Vegetable Glycerin • 1/8 CUP water • ½ TSP. Vitamin E Oil • 5 drops of Lavender Essential Oil • Container with lid • Small mixing bowl • Hand Blender	• Thoroughly blend ingredients in mixing bowl. • Transfer mixture into container. • Allow to set in cool place. • Store any remaining gel in your refrigerator.

GELATIN HAIR GEL	DIRECTIONS
• 1 TBSP. Unflavored Gelatin • ½ CUP. Of Hot Water • 8 oz. container with lid • ½ TSP. Vitamin E Oil • Stirring utensil	• Pour steaming hot water and all other ingredients into the container and stir. • Allow to set in cool place. • Store any remaining gel in your refrigerator.

This commandment will be a constant point of reference in this book because it reveals the foundation of what your hair products should consist of, as well as, multiple recipe choices for every hair product that you will need to care for your hair. If you chose to buy your hair products already packaged and created for you, this commandment will serve as a checklist for you to understand which hair products you can consider for purchase. Also, if you want to make some or all of your hair care products yourself, you can test the recipes given to decide what works best for your styling and hair care needs. Any recipes given in this commandment shall be used with your discretion in mind because everyone has different hair needs as well as a tolerance to certain ingredients used.

In the next commandment, COMMANDMENT VI, we will walk step by step through the process of caring for your natural hair now that you have been equipped with an ingredient checklist as well as your own homemade hair product recipes!

COMMANDMENT VI

THY HAIR SHALL REST ON THE SEVENTH DAY

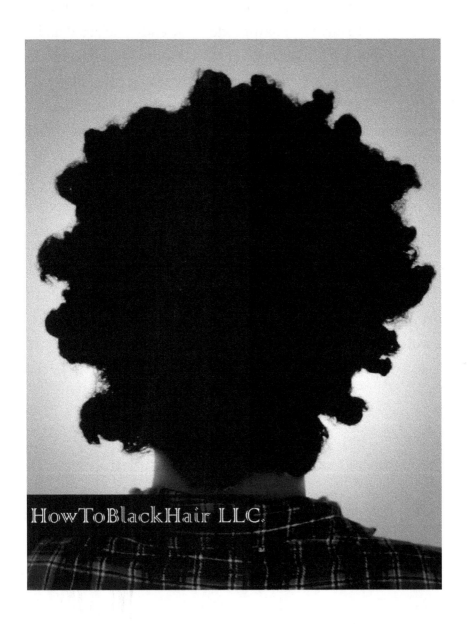

INTRODUCTION TO COMMANDMENT VI

YOUR HAIR SHALT ALWAYS RECEIVE ROYAL TREATMENT

Your hair shalt always receive royal treatment and everyone can experience such with their hair if they so desire. There is a misconception that caring for natural hair is very expensive because of the product arsenal that you need to have, in order to maintain healthy hair. The same can be applied to those who choose to chemically relax their hair because they also need to have a variety of products on hand to maintain healthy hair as well. Having healthy natural hair can be affordable, or not, depending on how much you choose to spend on your hair needs. Making your own homemade hair conditioner is usually cheaper and better for the environment while you can also choose to buy hair conditioner brands from hair salons only. The difference between those two options is not that one kind of conditioner will be better for your hair because that is not true; the only difference between the two options is preference. What may be affordable hair care products to you may not be affordable for someone else and vice versa so what really matters is that the products that you choose to use for hair care, gives you the desired affects that you were hoping for. Some who have natural hair love shampoos that produce a large amount of lather followed by a squeaky clean effect while others shy away from much lather and prefer their strands to feel thoroughly moisturized after a shampoo wash. Preference rules when it comes to treating your hair like royalty because you only want to give your hair what it needs, anything more or less can complicate your hair journey. When your hair feels drier than the usual, but you are not in need to shampoo, co-wash or deep condition your hair. If it is time to shampoo and you have had excessive dandruff or itching, wash more frequently and incorporate a few drops of Tea Tree Essential Oil into your products to control your dandruff and few drops of Lavender Essential Oil to soothe scalp inflammation as well. Another example as well for those who have unmanageable hair, even though you are probably consciously using quality products, is to continue to use your products while also only using distilled water as a water source for your hair. There are many ways to provide what your hair and scalp needs are besides the few examples that were previously stated. The best way to provide what your hair needs at all times, is to have a healthy hair care regimen so in this commandment, we will go step by step through the process of caring for your hair in order from Detangling, Co Washing, Shampooing, Deep Conditioning, Moisturizing, and Styling.

CREATING YOUR HAIR CARE MAINTENANCE ROUTINE

Your hair care routine is your most important routine because this is the grail of healthy hair care. Knowing how to properly detangle, how often to conditioner wash, shampoo, deep condition, moisturize, and style your hair equals success. Knowing how to perform each task, and when it is needed, will take away the majority of your worries about caring for your natural hair. The actual process of performing a natural hair care routine is what stops some individuals dead in their tracks because many of us have felt at one time or another, defeated by coily/kinky hair. This part of Commandment VI will walk you a step at a time to thoroughly assist you with your hair care routine.

DETANGLE (*to remove tangles, untangle*)

Detangle your hair before conditioner washing, shampooing, deep conditioning and styling. If you just want to conditioner wash or deep condition, detangle your hair before and style later.

Detangling For Styling	Detangling For; Cowashing, Shampooing, or Deep Conditioning
Step 1 Dampen or mist your hair with a water spray bottle. Step 2 Work moisturizer through your hair in manageable sections (about 4 -8 sections). Use hair clamps to assist you. Step 3 After applying moisturizer to all sections, wait at least 2- 5minutes to allow your hair to expand and become slippery for easier detangling. Step 4 Use your wide tooth comb to detangle a section, apply oil, and immediately set your hair in a desired fashion before moving on to the next section.	Step 1 Dampen your hair with a water spray bottle. Step 2 Work your detangling conditioner through your hair in manageable sections (about 4 -8 sections). Use hair clamps to assist you. Step 3 After applying moisturizer to all sections, wait at least 2- 5 minutes to allow your hair to expand and become slippery for easier detangling. Step 4 Use your wide tooth comb to detangle a section, two strand twist at the roots, and braid to the bottom of all sections. Proceed to the next step.

CONDITIONER WASH "COWASH" (*only conditioner washing to restore moisture*)

Cowash your hair if you need more moisture than just spritzing your hair. The frequency of cowashing your hair depends on your hair needs and it is typical to cowash once or twice a week.

Step 1 Dampen your hair with a water spray bottle.

Step 2 Work your detangling conditioner through your hair in manageable sections (about 4 -8 sections). Use hair clamps to assist you.

Step 3 After applying detangling conditioner to all sections, wait at least 2- 5 minutes to allow your hair to expand and become slippery for easier detangling.

Step 4 Use your wide tooth comb to detangle a section, two strand twist at the roots, and braid to the bottom of all sections, to perform the next step.

Steps 5 Thoroughly rinse all product from your hair with braided sections intact. Final rinse with the coolest water that you can stand, to close your cuticles.

Step 6 To keep your hair moisturized, layer your products on a section of hair at a time, in order of; moisturizer, oil, gel/pomade (optional).

> Step 7 Set your section of hair in a desired fashion before moving on to the next section.

SHAMPOO *(using a cleansing agent to wash your scalp and hair)*

Shampoo your hair to free your hair and scalp of natural buildup and/or product buildup. The frequency of shampooing your hair depends on your hair needs and it is typical to shampoo your hair once a week or every two weeks. Always detangle before shampooing. After shampooing your hair, always follow up with a deep condition.

> Step 1 Dampen your hair with a water spray bottle.
>
> Step 2 Work your detangling conditioner through your hair in manageable sections (about 4 -8 sections). Use hair clamps to assist you.
>
> Step 3 After applying detangling conditioner to all sections, wait at least 2- 5 minutes to allow your hair to expand and become slippery for easier detangling.
>
> Step 4 Use your wide tooth comb to detangle a section, two strand twist at the roots, and braid to the bottom of all sections, to perform the next step.

Step 5 Thoroughly rinse all product from your hair with braided sections intact, message shampoo on your scalp until clean and then focus on shampooing your hair.

Step 6 Thoroughly rinse all braided sections until there are no traces of shampoo. Do not final rinse with cool water because you want your cuticles open (raised) to allow the deep conditioner to penetrate easily.

Step 7 Follow up with a deep condition.

DEEP CONDITION *(using shaft penetrating ingredients to moisturize your hair for a designated amount of time)*

Deep condition your hair when your hair is experiencing more dryness than normal. The frequency of deep conditioning depends on your hair needs and it is typical to deep condition bi weekly or once a month. Use a plastic shower cap or a hooded dryer to allow warmth to open your hair strands even more for superb moisturization. Always deep condition your hair after shampooing to restore moisture within the hair shaft.

Step 1 Dampen your hair with a water spray bottle. Skip this step if your hair is already damp.

Step 2 Work your deep conditioner through your hair in manageable sections (about 4 -8 sections). Use hair clamps to assist you.

Step 3 After applying deep conditioner to all sections, wait at least 2- 5 minutes to allow your hair to expand and become slippery for easier detangling.

Step 4 Use your wide tooth comb to detangle a section, two strand twist at the roots, and braid to the bottom of all sections, to perform the next step.

Step 5 Cover your head with a plastic shower cap and wrap a towel around your head for about 30-45 minutes.

-OR-

Sit under a hooded dryer for 10-15 minutes while wearing a plastic shower cap.

Steps 6 Thoroughly rinse all product from your hair with braided sections intact.
Final rinse with the coolest water that you can stand, to close your cuticles.

Step 7 To keep your hair moisturized, layer your products on a section of hair at a time, in order of; moisturizer, oil, gel/pomade (optional).

Step 8 Set your section of hair in a desired fashion before moving on to the next section.

MOISTURIZE *(layering your hair with water, product, and oil to keep hair supple)*

Moisturize your hair when it is not quite fitting to cowash, deep condition, or shampoo your hair but you are in need of a subtle amount of moisture. The frequency of moisturization depends on your hair needs and it is typical to moisturize daily, every other day, or every 3 days.

Moisturize To Style Hair	Moisturize Without Styling Hair
Step 1 Dampen or mist your hair with a water spray bottle. Step 2 Work moisturizer through your hair in manageable sections (about 4 -8 sections). Use hair clamps to assist you. Step 3 After moisturizing, wait at least 2- 5 minutes to allow your hair to expand and become slippery for easier detangling/manipulation.	Step 1 Moisten or mist your hair with a water spray bottle. Step 2 Lightly coat your hands with your oil of choice and gently run your fingers and palms across your hair to seal in moisture. To preserve your style, don't run your fingers through your hair because this will cause frizz and loss of style definition.

Step 4 Use a wide tooth comb to detangle a section, apply oil, gel/pomade (optional) and immediately set your hair in a desired fashion before moving on to the next sections.	

STYLING *(fashioning your hair by manipulation)*

Styling your hair has an unlimited amount of choices so let your imagination take you to where you want your hair to be. You can choose to opt for a simple or elaborate hairstyle but keep in mind that the less manipulation required to keep your hair tidy, the less hair damage you will experience from wear and tear. You can style/reset your hair into another style immediately after detangling, cowashing, deep conditioning, and even moisturizing. You cannot style your hair after shampooing because remember, you have to follow up with a deep condition to restore moisture into your hair. Directions below are in the case of restyling your hair without experiencing a cowash or a deep condition.

Step 1 Work in manageable sections (about 4 -8 sections). Use hair clamps to assist you.

Hair Tip Working on damp hair will give your hair crisp definition while working on dry hair will give you soft definition. It is preferred to work on damp hair for gentler manipulation but if you want softer definition, lightly mist your hair instead of dampening it.

Step 2 After misting or dampening your hair with your moisturizer (preferably a liquid moisturizer), wait at least 2- 5 minutes to allow your hair to expand and become slippery for easier detangling.

Step 3 To keep your hair moisturized, layer your products on a section of hair at a time, in order of; moisturizer, oil, gel/pomade (optional).

Step 4 Set your section of hair in a desired fashion before moving on to the next section.

My Natural Hairstyling tutorial videos can be found on both of my YouTube channels

BlackWomenHair YouTube Channel
www.youtube.com/BlackWomenHair

HowToBlackHair YouTube Channel
www.youtube.com/HowToBlackHair

Every step within the healthy hair care regimen previously explored, is applicable for very tight curl patterns to very loose curl patterns. Two strand twisting your hair at your roots and braiding to the ends of your hair, section by section, allows room for you to cleanse your scalp with a cleanser/shampoo effectively without producing tangles. Because the ends of your sections are braided, this greatly prevents your hair from continuing to coil at the ends, which we know, creates single strand knots that have to be trimmed later. Twisting the roots and braiding to the ends is highly suggested for Type 4 Hair and some tighter patterned Type 3 Hair as well. If you absolutely think that it is unnecessary to work section by section, twisting your roots and braiding to the ends of your hair, then by all means, perform your hair regimen with free flowing hair. Following the techniques presented in this healthy hair care regimen, will keep your hair healthy and in prime condition for all hair types and textures.

Next, in COMMANDMENT VII, we will explore a very controversial mindset within the hair community that can be very discouraging to individuals new to natural hair. If you are not careful, you could very well find yourself adopting this cookie cutter complex as well.

COMMANDMENT VII

THOU SHALT NOT BECOME A NATURAL HAIR NAZI

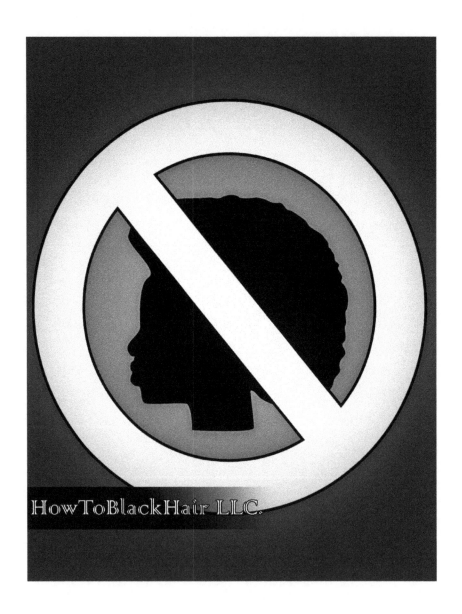

INTRODUCTION TO COMMANDMENT VII

HAVING NATURAL HAIR DOES NOT MAKE YOU AFROCENTRIC

Having natural hair does not make you Afrocentric nor should it pressure you to discover your" true self" on a journey towards your "homeland". A very prominent forethought when deciding to finally embrace and accept the hair that grows out of your head naturally, has always been the vivid image of proud black people wearing gigantic afros with their fists raised high in the air. Some of you may not have had this image painted in your mind but many people have. I have witnessed countless influences on the internet alone, promoting natural hair as a journey back to your ancestral roots. I root for those who have allowed their hair to inspire them to blossom into the person they have always wanted to become. Some women accept their natural hair while simultaneously adopting more of a holistic lifestyle consisting of usually; a cleaner diet, herbal remedies, and spirituality. In some cases, those who chose to embrace their natural hair, project their intellect upon the natural hair community out of a place of pride and self-righteousness. When you are not careful, your passion for natural hair can suffocate you and make your lifestyle more complicated than what it needs to be. Swearing only by natural organic ingredients, unmanipulated hair, and that extensions represent self-hate, has turned casual online hair forum discussions upside down! There are already enough external hair pressures plastered on magazine covers and flaunted about on the red carpet, and still some people are being cut down about having true natural hair? By default, natural hair is hair that is free of chemical relaxers so if someone has hair with heat damage/heat trains, wears weaves, or has color, are they unnatural? So far, many commandments have been pressed upon you in regards to taking care of your natural hair but never do I expect you to take the advice given and become completely obsessive about it. Being consumed with a legality about natural hair will have you torn between doing "what's right" and what you truly want to do with your hair. These commandments are here to give you a strong, solid foundation for healthy natural hair care, not to enslave you or slap your wrist for doing things that work but may not be standard. Steer clear from those who guilt you about the things that work for you and your hair because it is not standard. Even to those who are chemically relaxing their hair and have decided to read this book, if you are happy with your hair and you do not want to change a thing, do not be pressured to. Let your hair be a representation of how you want to represent yourself to the world, not matter your hair type or texture. Now, let us dig deeper and journey through the extreme views of various hair topics.

EMBRACING YOUR UNMANIPULATED

CURL PATTERN

Of course we all want to do things right when it comes to our hair or at least give our hair the best treatment that we can, with the abilities that we have. That is why low manipulation styles like mini twists, braid outs, and afro puffs remain simple go to styles for many new and seasoned naturals. These hair styles can help your hair reach its greatest potential in health and length since heat or harsh chemicals are not required to achieve beautiful results. Even though these styles exude confidence and flatter natural hair, some people may have problems with this and those people are usually called Natural Hair Nazis.

Natural Hair Nazi: a die-hard natural hair enthusiast that labels others as a true natural based off product choices and/or styling options, beyond the undisputed universal definition of having natural hair.

Natural Hair: hair that is not chemically/permanently treated to change the texture/curl pattern that naturally grows from your scalp.

According to some Natural Hair Nazis, always manipulating your hair to achieve a hairstyle is not being a true natural because a true natural should accept their hair as is without manually manipulating it for a desired shape and look. Do not be bothered by this train of thought that assumes you dislike your natural hair because you always have to manipulate it into a style to make it acceptable unto you. Taking this logic as far as it goes even discriminates against those who wear picked afros, traditional locs or sister locs, since manipulation is required. This thinking encourages free formed locs. It is only fitting that every natural hair nazi, with this belief, should have free form locs because they deem constant manipulated hairstyles as a way of showing that you do not like your curl pattern.

Wearing your hair constantly manipulated to take on a style of your choice does not make you any more or less natural than the next person. In fact, wearing styles like mini twists and braids are very helpful for those who live busy lives and cannot cater to a twist out or braid out daily. Listening to the advice of sporting unmanipulated hair is unnecessary. Now, let us discuss the next topic with still much controversy to this day, hair products.

THE TALK ON HAIR PRODUCTS

There are an unlimited amount of choices to choose from when it comes to hair products. Just think about how many hair products are on the shelves of your local drugstore promising to fix a number of hair issues like split ends, thin frizzy hair, and color fading? Within the natural hair community, Natural Hair Nazis bring home the point that only using natural ingredients in your hair products are best for your hair. Also, another point made, in relation to hair extensions, is that hair weaves/extensions cause permanent hair damage and it also shows that you shame your natural hair because of your choice to cover your hair with extensions. This rationale should be considered to a degree when thinking about the quality of ingredients in your hair products and the risk of hair loss when it comes to wearing hair extensions.

HAIR CARE PRODUCTS

When it comes to hair care products, your typical Natural Hair Nazi will tell you how important it is to only use natural ingredients in all of your hair care products. This reason is backed by the notion alone that you should only use natural products to provide the best for your natural hair. This notion would deserve more applause if it was coming from a place of using natural products because it is biodegradable and therefore, better for the environment. Assuming that only using products that are 100% natural are best for healthy natural hair, leaves out those with healthy hair, who use products that are not 100% natural. Previously in COMMANDMENT V, you have been advised on the ingredients you want to have in your hair products and those that you want to stay away from. The list of ingredients that you have been forewarned to stay away from, are unnecessary and damaging to your hair. Consider the fact that some chemicals derived from other ingredients are still considered a natural ingredient by some. For instance, you can derive sodium lauryl sulfate from coconut oil (which is a cleansing agent you want to avoid using on your hair). What makes this cleansing agent bad are the effects that it has on your hair, not that it is a chemical derived from a natural ingredient. To the person who lives in an area with hard water, using a stronger cleansing agent in their shampoo is ideal for the health of their hair. In relation to the pressing emphasis placed on only using natural products, I wonder if these die hard enthusiasts make sure to only eat 100% natural organic foods since what goes into the body, is definitely more important than how the outside of the body looks?

HAIR EXTENSIONS

Using hair extensions to enhance your beauty no longer brings shame to women today like it did in the past because now, hair is treated like an accessory. Depending on the type of weave and extension that you chose to wear, this can represent a level of social status that you may or may not already have. The problem that many Natural Hair Nazis have with hair extensions is that number one, they say it eventually leads to traction alopecia and number two, it is used to cover the shame that you may have for your natural hair. Both of these reasons against wearing extensions/weaves do hold some weight to it but this is dependent upon by the wearer, not the judgmental assumption given by die hards.

Traction Alopecia: traumatic (or repeated) stress (outside forces) on your hair and scalp that leads to hair loss. This can be seen in the form of a bald patch/patches or a receding hairline.

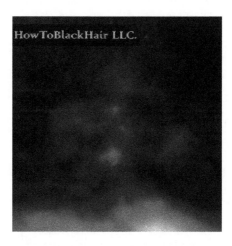

Extreme close up of traction alopecia

To clear the air once and for all, weaves/extensions do not cause traction alopecia. The reason why so many people may think that this form of alopecia is caused by this is because developing this alopecia happens frequently with those who wear hair extensions. You can also begin to develop traction alopecia from constantly scratching/rubbing a certain area of your scalp along with constantly gathering your real hair into tight ponytails. The very nature of weaves and extensions helps you to retain length and keep your hair protected from daily manipulation. When extensions are not installed properly and comfortably, you will lose hair and in most cases, your hairline will start to recede. At this time, many pictures have surfaced on the internet of a famous super model experiencing traction alopecia from what is assumed to be unnecessary tension being placed on her hairline. This person could have had an internal issue that has led her to losing her hair but the visual appearance of her hair loss, is very typical of what someone's hairline starts to look like after a repeat of installs that were too stressful on the hair and scalp. Wearing extensions/weaves are very helpful for naturals who may not be able to style their hair often and, it is also a great way of transitioning to the length that you would like to have. Also, the joys of weaves and extensions allow you to experiment with a different cut, color, or style without changing the state of your real hair. If hair extensions and weaves are installed properly, comfortably, and your real hair is cared for underneath, there are no reasons as to why extensions should not be considered optional with natural hair.

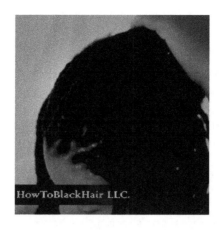

HowToBlackHair LLC.

A big discussion highlighted by many Natural Hair Nazis is that those with natural hair, only truly wear extensions/weaves out of a place of self-hate. This belief cannot be held true for anyone who chooses to either rarely wear weaves or obsessively wear weaves. It is impossible to truly judge the motives behind why someone may choose to always wear hair extensions unless the person decides to admit that they in fact, dislike their natural hair. Even if someone with natural hair professes this to the world, you should care less and spare your judgment! If you must speak on this, it is best to uplift the person and encourage them in the fact that they are beautiful and their hair rocks without hair extensions. That person who always wears weaves could be doing it for the sake of their job, out of convenience, or to cover up whatever shame they may have in relation to the state of their hair. That person has to live with their hair, no one else does. If you are someone who feels as though you cannot live without extensions, that is your decision so do what is best for you. If you are that same person but you want to live without needing hair extensions, then work on learning to love and accept your hair for what is, no matter what anyone says or how you internally feel about your natural hair. The problem with the thinking of Natural Hair Nazis, in relation to this topic, is that they think truly accepting natural hair is forever saying no to weaves and extensions and if you do not, you have not accepted yourself. That belief has taken hair styling so far out of context, along with others, that it leaves me to wonder how these die hard enthusiasts choose to wear their hair because according to their "laws", there are not much options! I leave you on this note, let your hair extensions "extend" the beauty that you already have and if you only feel beautiful with hair extensions, dig down deep on why you feel that way and learn to accept and love yourself as you are.

In the next commandment, COMMANDMENT VIII, we will elaborate more on how wearing hair extensions can be of help to you when working with the versatility of your natural hair or transitioning hair.

COMMANDMENT VIII

WEAVES ARE NOT THY ENEMY

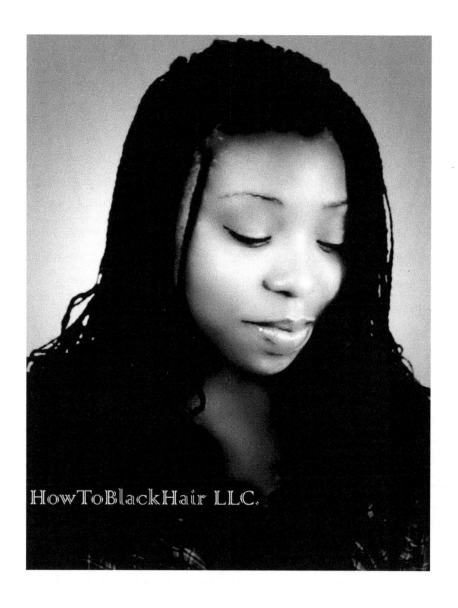

INTRODUCTION TO COMMANDMENT VIII

THEY SAY DIAMONDS ARE A GIRLS BEST FRIEND

They say diamonds are a girl's best friend but in all honesty, weaves are! Extensions and weaves have been crossing racial boundaries since its existence. For example, if a white/Caucasian woman is wearing extensions, their favorite choice of hair would probably be predominate of these various options; cold fusions, hot fusions, or clip ins. When you think about an ethnic woman, her weave/extensions of choice are predominately these various options; sew ins, lace wigs, quick weaves, and braids. Of course all women do not wear weaves or extensions but, we cannot ignore the fact that more women everyday are converting into an occasional wearer of hair pieces while some become complete weavaholics!

Weaveaholic: an extension/weave obsessed individual that loves to wear many different kinds of textures and curl patterns. It is typical for this individual to constantly change the look of their hair.

Being a weaveaholic is nothing to be ashamed of, do what brings you joy as long as it does not involve hurting yourself or others. Extensions can become a problem when they come before your well-being or/and the well-being of others under your care. In some cases, some women have chosen their hair over paying a utility bill and in other cases, I have even personally noticed women prioritizing their hair over the way that their children are fashioned before going out into public. This very type of weaveaholic is mindboggling because in any case scenario, this individual rationalizes their weave/extensions as the top tier of important matters. This alone is a different conversation because there is a deeper problem underneath the superficial reverence that they have for their hair.

It is ok to love weaves and extensions if it is within your means and you are able to wear different kinds of looks without sacrificing any area of your life. As a teenager, I always restyled my hair every two weeks so I would go to my local beauty supply store and scan the isles to capture my next look. Sometimes I wanted to have long and flowy hair with wispy flipped ends, have a curly bob, or rock wavy hair with an extreme deep side part. If I could not afford to try a more expensive brand of hair, I did not buy it. If there were sales on a certain kinds of extensions because of a surplus of inventory, I would stock up on different curl patterns and colors to experiment with other options. Next, I will show you different types of weaves/extensions styles you can choose to wear with your natural/transitioning hair to give you more styling options.

HAIRSTYLES FOR NATURAL AND

TRANSITIONING HAIR

This section of COMMANDMENT VIII will showcase many possible styles that you can wear with your natural and/or transitioning hair. If you want, consider the styling options portrayed that allows you to conceal all of your hair or, give you the ability to blend with your leave out.

Leave Out: leaving out a section of your real hair to conceal over the bind/attachment of your weave and or extensions.

Any hair styling options featured can be found in detailed hair tutorial videos, step by step, on both of my YouTube channels.

BlackWomenHair YouTube Channel
www.youtube.com/BlackWomenHair

HowToBlackHair YouTube Channel
www.youtube.com/HowToBlackHair

You can also search any style you would like to see on my website: www.Howtoblackhair.com

Without further ado, each style shown in picture form will go in the order of difficulty and start with the name of the style, a brief description of how to achieve the style, how to find my step by step video hair tutorial of my style, and picture(s) of the style.

Cornrow Braids on Natural Hair

These braids are also referred to as french braids, scalp braids or small dutch braids.

Your hair is first detangled and sectioned accordingly. You will part and plait three strands of your hair at a time while occasionally adding more of your hair unto a leg of your braid.

For this style, search my YouTube channels and website for "cornrows"

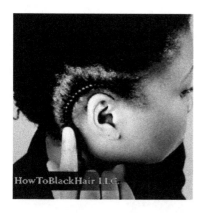 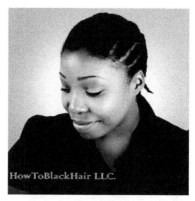

Crochet/Latch Hook Braids

This style is called latch hook braids or crochet braids.

Your hair is first detangled and sectioned accordingly. Hair will be braided in two layers of cornrows. The cornrows in the back of your head are half the amount of cornrows in the front of your head. For example, 12 cornrows in the front, 6 cornrows in the back. Braiding hair is then weaved underneath all cornrow braids with a beader or a latch hook tool.

For this style, search my YouTube channels and website for "crochet braids"

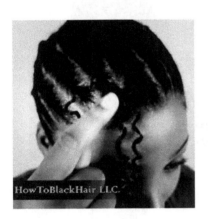 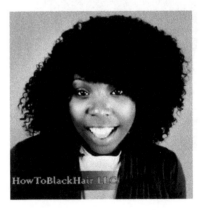

Senegalese/Rope Twists

This style is called senegalese twists or rope twists.

Your hair is first detangled and sectioned accordingly. Braiding hair is sectioned and divided into two. The middle point of a portion of braiding hair is pressed against the scalp, as each section twists in opposite directions. As each section continues to twist in opposite directions of one another, the twists overlap one another.

For this style, search my YouTube channels and website for "rope twists".

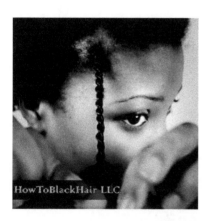 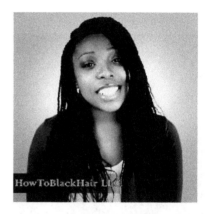

Cornrow Braids with Extensions

Your hair is first detangled and sectioned accordingly. An amount of braiding hair will be split into two parts; one part is two-thirds of your original amount and the other part is one-third of your original amount. The one-third section will fold over the two-thirds section to form three equal legs to your braiding hair. As the braiding hair is fashioned around your fingers, you will proceed to braid with the cornrow technique while constantly incorporating your braiding hair.

For this style, search my YouTube channels and website for "cornrow extensions".

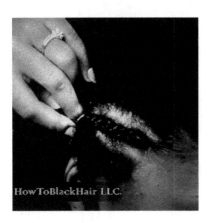
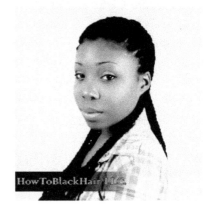

Kinky Twists

Your hair is first detangled and sectioned accordingly. An amount of braiding hair will be split into two parts; one part is two-thirds of your original amount and the other part is one-third of your original amount. The one-third section will fold over the two-thirds section to form three equal legs to your braiding hair. As the braiding hair is fashioned around your fingers, you will gather all of your real hair onto one leg of your braiding hair. Braid a couple of times away from your scalp, split the middle leg of your extension hair, and two strand twist to the very bottom. For the signature look, the ends of your kinky twist will be rolled in cold wave rods and dipped in hot water.

For this style, search my YouTube channels and website for "kinky twist"

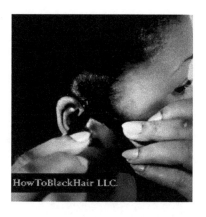 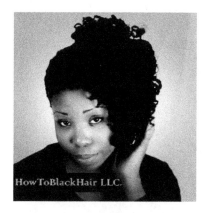

Yarn Braids / Genie Locs

This style is called yarn braids or genie locs. They are also incorrectly referred to as fake dreadlocs. Fake locs require a different technique and can be achieved with yarn or braiding hair.

Your hair is first detangled and sectioned accordingly. With a couple of strands of acrylic yarn, you will adopt the similar technique of preparing braiding hair like individual braids. With the acrylic yarn fashioned around your fingers, you will gather all of your real hair onto one leg of your section of acrylic yarn, and braid away from the scalp. Braid all the way down until you are left with about an inch of distance from finishing. Tie multiple knots at the bottom and snip any leftover yarn. A candle or cigarette lighter is commonly used to seal the ends but I highly discourage it.

For this style, search my YouTube channels and website for "yarn braids"

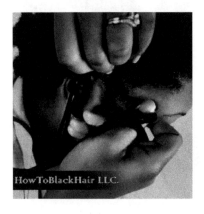 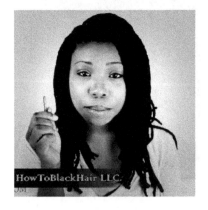

Patra Braids/Jumbo Braids

This style is called patra braids or jumbo braids. These braids are typically double the size of box braids even though they are achieved with the exact same braiding technique.

Your hair is first detangled and sectioned accordingly. An amount of braiding hair will be split into two parts; one part is two-thirds of your original amount and the other part is one-third of your original amount. The one-third section will fold over the two-thirds section to form three equal legs to your braiding hair. As the braiding hair is fashioned around your fingers, you will gather all of her real hair onto one leg of your braiding hair. Braid all the way down to the bottom. To seal the ends, you will dip them in hot water.

For this style, search my YouTube channels and website for "Patra Braids"

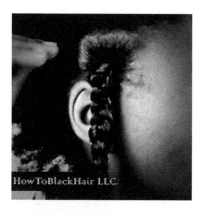 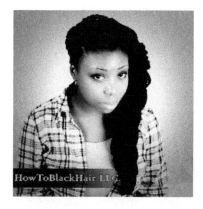

Single Braids/Box Braids

This style is called single braids or box braids. It is also referred to as poetic justice braids, Janet braids or Solange braids. These braids are typically half the size of patra braids even though they are achieved with the exact same braiding technique.

Your hair is first detangled and sectioned accordingly. An amount of braiding hair will be split into two parts; one part is two-thirds of your original amount and the other part is one-third of your original amount. The one-third section will fold over the two-thirds section to form three equal legs to your braiding hair. As the braiding hair is fashioned around your fingers, you will gather all of your real hair onto one leg of your braiding hair. Braid all the way down to the bottom. To seal the ends, you will dip them in hot water.

For this style, search my YouTube channels and website for "Box Braids on Natural Hair"

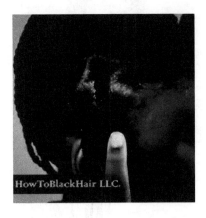 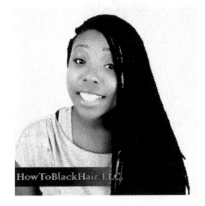

Zillion/Micro Braids

This style is called micro braids or zillion braids. These braids are typically half the size of single braids even though they are achieved with the exact same braiding technique.

Your hair is first detangled and sectioned accordingly. An amount of braiding hair will be split into two parts; one part is two-thirds of your original amount and the other part is one-third of your original amount. The one-third section will fold over the two-thirds section to form three equal legs to your braiding hair. As the braiding hair is fashioned around your fingers, you will gather all of your real hair onto one leg of your braiding hair. Braid all the way down to the bottom. To seal the ends, you will dip them in hot water or curl the ends with the kinky twist technique.

For this style, search my YouTube channels and website for "Micro Braids"

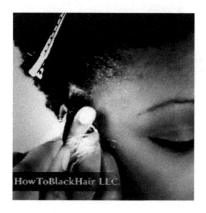
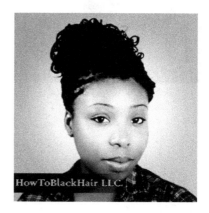

Full Wig

Choose any kind of curl pattern, texture or color with your choice of *weave because this hairstyle requires no leave out.*

Your hair is first detangled and sectioned accordingly. Braid all of your hair in cornrows or twists, cornrows are preferred. You will sew in your hair weave unto a wig cap, on a manikin head that is the same size as your head. After leaving a small circle at the top of the wig cap, you will sew into that space your handmade closure piece. After placing the wig onto your head, you will style it to your liking.

For this style, search my YouTube channels and website for

"Full Wig"

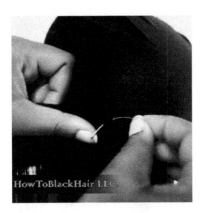
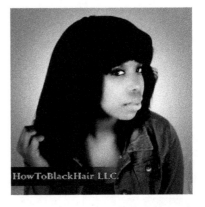

U Part Wig

Use weave that matches your natural curl pattern. You can also buy hair weave that matches the pattern of your braid out, twist out, or even your afro if that is the pattern you would like to wear to match with your weave.

A U part section of your hair will be preserved as your leave out. The rest of your hair will be braided. You will have a cornrow braid that goes all the way around the perimeter of your hairline and leave out area while the rest of your hair will be braided to the back in cornrows. You will sew in your hair weave unto a wig cap, on a manikin head that is the same size as your head. After leaving a u-shaped opening near the front of the wig, cut off any remaining cap and sew the wig unto your head. After placing the wig onto your head, you will blend your leave out with your weave and further style your wig to your liking.

For this style, search my YouTube channels and website for

"U Part Wig"

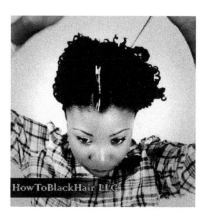 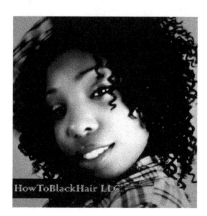

L Part Wig

Use weave that matches your natural curl pattern. You can also buy hair weave that matches the pattern of your braid out, twist out, or even your afro if that is the pattern you would like to wear to match with your weave.

An L part section of your hair will be preserved as your leave out. The rest of your hair will be braided. You will have a cornrow braid that goes all the way around the perimeter of your hairline and leave out area while the rest of your hair will be braided to the back in cornrows. You will sew in your hair weave unto a wig cap, on a manikin head that is the same size as your head. After leaving an L shaped opening near the front of the wig, cut off any remaining cap and sew the wig unto your head. After placing the wig onto your head, you will blend your leave out with your weave and further style your wig to your liking.

For this style, search my YouTube channels and website for

"L Part Wig"

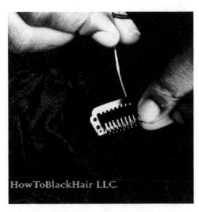
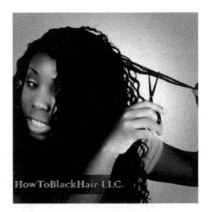

Invisible Part Sew In

Choose any kind of curl pattern, texture or color with your choice of *weave because this hairstyle requires no leave out.*

A wide u part section of your hair will have an even amount of cornrow braids facing away from one another. You will have a cornrow braid that goes all the way around the perimeter of your hairline while the rest of your hair will be braided in cornrows. You will sew in your hair weave onto your braids in a u shaped fashion without sewing onto the base where the invisible part will be. With very small pieces of weave, you will sew it onto each braid, of the base of the invisible part area, one by one. After leaving a small circle at the top near your invisible part base, you will sew into that space your handmade closure piece. After sewing all of your weave, style your look to your liking.

For this style, search my YouTube channels and website for "Invisible Part Sew In"

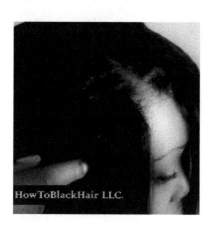 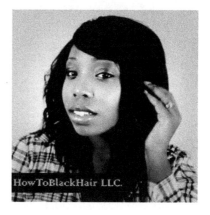

Net Weave Full Sew In

Choose any kind of curl pattern, texture or color with your choice of weave because this hairstyle requires no leave out.

You will begin by braiding a cornrow braid all the way around the perimeter of your hairline while the rest of your hair will be braided in cornrows. You will then sew your weaving net onto your perimeter braid with my sewing technique. Sew your weave in a circular fashion and leave a small circle at the top of your head for your handmade closure. After sewing in all of your weave, style your sew in to your liking.

For this style, search my YouTube channels and website for "Net Weave Sew In"

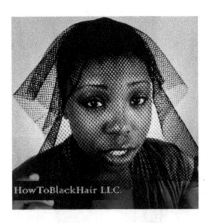

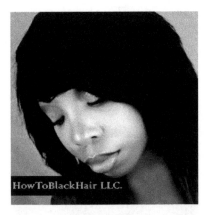

In this commandment, you have been given a vast amount of weave and extension hairstyles that you can wear with your natural hair. All styling options are also applicable if you are transitioning onto natural hair as well. Wearing extensions is an optional styling choice if you want to use it in place of a desirable length and/or thickness, or, if you want to try different looks before making any drastic changes to your hair. Also, when searching for my various styles depicted in this commandment, make sure you are subscribed to both of my YouTube channels, HowToBlackHair and BlackWomenHair. You will receive hair tutorials that I occasionally release because upon reading this book, you will miss many hair tutorial videos if you are not subscribed. If you are having troubles navigating or want to make sure that you are able to connect with me effectively, my email is howtoblackhair.breannarutter@gmail.com

In the next commandment, COMMANDMENT VIIII, we will discuss the topic of loving thy relaxed neighbors.

COMMANDMENT VIIII

LOVE THY RELAXED NEIGHBORS

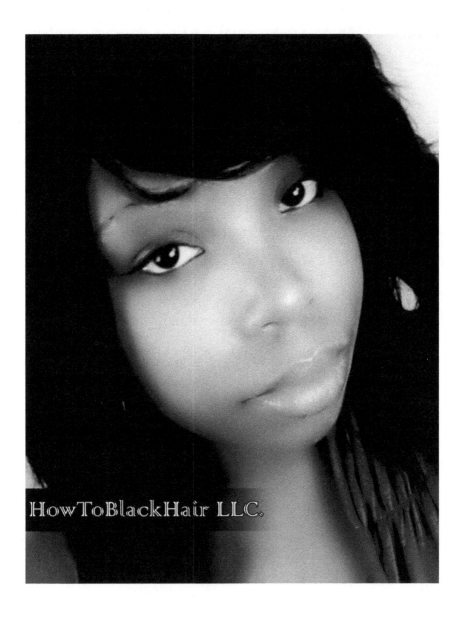

HowToBlackHair LLC.

INTRODUCTION TO COMMANDMENT VIIII

I ALWAYS REMEMBER SEEING HER PERFECT BROWN CURLS

I always remember seeing her perfect brown curls cascading down her back whether she had a good hair day or a bad one, I could not tell the difference between the two. My classmate and I would always small talk in 6th grade gym class and I remember her complaining to me one day about how bad her hair was because her ponytail kept frizzing. I said, "What? You're sure you're having a bad hair day?" She said "Yes! Look at my hair ugh!" I could not see past her long bouncy curls and as time passed during the hot days in gym class, her sleek curly ponytail become more wild and bold. As much as she hated her hair that day, I was wishing I could have it. She was biracial, Hispanic and Black, and we were very similar. We were similar in size, height, color, wittiness, even down to a similar laid back casual style of dress! What bothered me the most was that through so many similarities, her hair was still vastly different than mine and I longed to have her hair. I never felt ill towards her because of her hair; I just wanted hair like hers. I loved brushing her hair and occasionally braiding a cute patch of designed cornrow braids for her just because. She had the only type of natural hair I remember seeing probably because that is what I thought natural hair was. With the mind of a preteen, I thought natural hair was only what I now know as Type 3 hair. I rarely ever seen those who had type 4 hair and if I did, it was only new growth waiting to receive a touch up from a chemical relaxer. Seeing my roots unrelaxed did not sicken me like it did for others, it scared me! I had no idea how to work with two different textures of hair and I did not want to bear the shame of being looked down upon for my unrelaxed roots so sadly, I stayed enslaved to the "creamy crack".

I said all this to give insight on the mentality that I had being a relaxed child and that there are so many different reasons as to why someone chooses to relax their hair. Some may be closed minded to the different types of textures and curls existing beyond their horizon or, may not have had much exposure to diverse kinds of hair. At a young age, natural hair that was not in the Type 3 range was considered too kinky and nappy to deal with so if you did not have "mixed hair", being natural was a lonely path you would shamelessly walk on by yourself. Ignorance can bring on a lot of hurt and pain because your reality of what is, and what's not, can be very offensive and hurtful to others for multiple reasons. This commandment does not promote a pro natural/ anti-relaxed mentality, this commandment is here to open our eyes to how we should be mindful of how we respect and communicate with someone who chooses to wear natural hair or not.

ADDRESSING CREAMY CRACK INDIVIDUALS

Creamy Crack: The slang name/term for a chemical relaxer.

Companies are paying much attention to the sweeping influence that natural hair has within the African American community. It is rumored that between the year of 2011-2012, chemical relaxer sales declined by 17%. The significance of the percentage of sales must mean much because many familiar ethnic hair brands are now starting to incorporate hair care products catered specifically towards natural hair.

Aside from the business aspect of cashing in on natural hair, a lot of chemically relaxed individuals are chiming in on those who wear natural hair. There is a prevalent argument taking place between the relaxed and non-relaxed on YouTube videos and websites catered towards ethnic hair. The problem is not an indifference of opinion in regards to how someone chooses to manipulate and care for their hair, the problem is the way that some chemically relaxed individuals convey their ideas towards those who have natural hair. Often, I have personally witnessed on a forum, or comments on a video/website, of a relaxed individual cutting down another who chooses not to relax their hair. Some individuals who relax their hair assume that someone with natural hair is lazy and that their hair is always uncared for. Just as much trial and error, research, and patience, goes into natural hair similarly to someone who decides to have relaxed hair. Relaxed and Natural individuals predominately want the same results for their hair such as; having healthy, manageable long hair.

The best way to address someone who is cutting you down is to respond with love. I know it may be difficult because it is in our nature to defend ourselves against someone who is offending you but two people offending each other can justify their ill response toward one another. If a relaxed individual is putting you down about having natural hair, respond with respect or ignore them.

For instance, someone once told me, "Girl, your hair is too nappy!" I could have responded by saying, "You're ignorant, I chose to wear my "real hair" instead of being ashamed by relaxing it and straightening it like you!" Responding that way assumes that the person straightens or relaxes their hair and that they do so out of shame. She may have had natural hair that wasn't as "nappy" as mine is. My response to that ill comment will not give her an open change of mind; it will open the opportunity for her to be offensive once again. The best way to respond is to say, "That's your opinion, I like it that my natural hair is really thick and kinky". Or you can simply ignore that person and move on. Does moving on allow that person to win? No. Moving on makes you the better person in the end. It is your choice whether or not that conversation is worth your time and attention, if you do chose to converse, do so with love and respect.

BE ENCOURAGING TO OTHERS, NOT DEMEANING

In the beginning of this commandment, the focus was on helping those with natural hair understand how to address aggressive individuals that relax their hair. In this section we will focus on the way that some naturals treat those who chose to chemically relax their hair.

The offensive treatment between those with natural hair and chemically relaxed hair seems to be of an equal force. Depending on which side of the fence you stand on, you may feel like your opposite clashes with a greater force than that of your counterparts. In other words, if you have natural hair, you may feel as though those who have chemically relaxed hair respond with more hostility towards you, than naturals do towards those who relax. The topic of hair within the African American community will always be a sensitive one, so striking the nerve of another on the topic of hair, is never a hard task to do.

For example, a stigma that follows the thoughts of some with natural hair is that those who chemically relax their hair do not accept themselves because they do not accept the hair that they were naturally born with. This type of attitude towards those who chemically relax their hair is very offensive and unnecessary. Someone who chooses to chemically relax their hair may feel as though their hair suits their lifestyle. Even if the root of their choice to chemically relax is one of a dislike for their natural hair, that's their decision and their choice should not encourage your voicing of disapproval.

Every person that relaxes their hair isn't looking to be converted so pressing your natural hair beliefs on those who relax is coming from a place of much pride and self-righteousness. It is a fact that a curious mind asks questions so do not assume that someone wants to know why you have chosen not relax your hair unless they ask you directly. It hurts just the same to see someone with natural hair criticize someone who relaxes their hair; everyone's hair decision is their own.

Bombarding those who chemically relax their hair with information that no one asked for can be just as offensive as cutting someone down for chemically relaxing their hair. Trying to come to someone's rescue who does not need to be saved is very annoying, be encouraging if someone who relaxes is looking for your encouragement and continue to project a positive and uplifting voice within the hair community.

In the beginning of this commandment, we discussed the topic of addressing creamy crack individuals. Sometimes there are those people who can never seem to understand why you have committed to having natural hair and that is ok. The hair you wear on your head is not to be in accordance to another's belief nor should you expect them to respect your hair choice either. Also, there are times when the response of someone who relax can make you so upset, that you want to fire right back. The best thing to do is to be the better person by responding with love, or simply ignoring what they have said and move on.

Towards the end of this commandment, we discussed the topic of being encouraging and not demeaning. Overexerting your natural beliefs and thoughts of assumptions onto those who relax their hair can be just as overwhelming and offensive. Someone who relaxes their hair does not need to be converted onto the natural side. The same goes for those who have natural hair as well.

In the next commandment, COMMANDMENT X, we will talk about loving and accepting thine own hair.

COMMANDMENT X

ABOVE ALL ELSE, LOVE AND ACCEPT THINE OWN HAIR

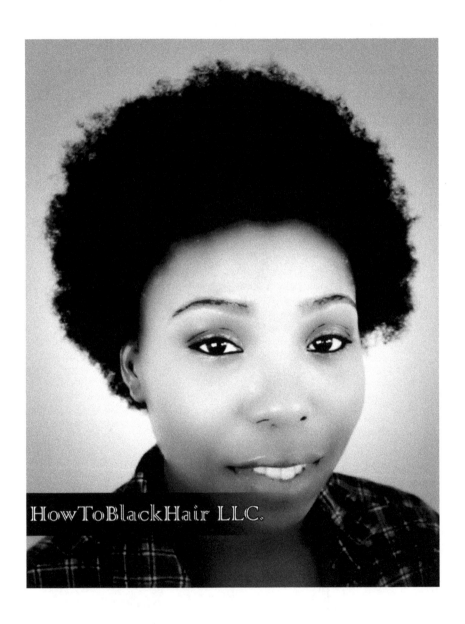

INTRODUCTION TO COMMANDMENT X

IT'S EASY TO REFLECT ON THE THINGS THAT YOU DON'T LIKE TO SEE

It's easy to reflect on the things that you don't like to see rather than the things that you do like to see when looking in the mirror. That mirror you occasionally glance at occasionally throughout the day shows you a direct reflection of yourself, but not a direct reflection of what you internalize.

When I was a teenager I went through the whole body conscious phase that everyone else went through. Friends and family would look at me and say that I looked good but when I looked in the mirror, I didn't see what everyone else saw. It's ok to go through that in life because being body conscious helps you to realize what you want to see within yourself and this is healthy, in most cases. In extreme cases, a lot of teenage children will have such a warped view of their body that they will starve themselves of the food and nutrition their growing body needs. I never fit into that category but I could see how things could spiral in that direction if I constantly obsessed over my imperfections.

In relation to hair, we can obsess over its image in similar ways. Usually new naturals are extremely anxious on finding out what their hair type is. It becomes an obsession even though there may not be much natural roots present to determine where they lie on the curl spectrum. Comparing our bodies to others that we reverence in some way also applies in similar ways to how we can obsessively compare our hair to others. Having a "curl crush" can inspire you to reach new lengths and it also can easily lead you to wishing you had hair just like theirs.

Cherish the fact that the hair that you have on your head is unique and no one else can have hair just like you. No matter who you are or what your hair type is, there is someone out there in the world that covets your hair also.

This commandment is focused on giving you the encouragement that you need to love and accept thine own hair, above all others.

LET YOUR HAIR REFLECT YOUR LIFESTYLE

The saying that goes, "Everyone can't have natural hair" is true in the context that I am going to explain. Natural hair is not for those who do not want to learn how to care for it and cater it into their lifestyle. If you expect natural hair to thrive on its own without applying the correct techniques and using the right products, then expect to endure exhausting self-inflicted consequences for doing so. Having natural hair can be easier or more difficult depending on the way an individual views the maintenance but in all honesty, natural hair and relaxed hair can equate to a similarity of the energy taken in maintenance.

When understanding exactly what you should do to allow your natural hair to reflect your lifestyle, start with implementing an easy regimen. Do you work full time? Play sports? Have children? Work from home? There are so many different kinds of lifestyles that we all have, we are all different from one another so it is only natural that our hair maintenance process will differ as well. If you do not have a demanding job, your hair in any natural state, manipulated or not, can fit into your lifestyle. On the opposite end, if you are a busy college student, wearing a braid out every single day can become very time consuming when you don't have much time to give. Wearing natural hair in this situation, as well as any other kind of busy situation, is possible by wearing hairstyles that do not require you to manipulate your hair often (like mini twists) and also by wearing extensions and weaves as protective styles.

Protective Style: a hairstyle that requires low manipulation with usually concealed ends. It is also free of harsh chemicals and heat. The degree of what is a protective style or not, varies from person to person. For example, two strand twists would be viewed as a protective style and not a twist out even though, both styles fit this very description.

The maintenance of your hair should never take time away from the things that are most important to you. If you like to have your natural hair colored, consider highlights first for easier maintenance. Committing to a full head of color only becomes a problem if you cannot commit to constantly deep conditioning your hair, occasional color rinses and regularly touching up your roots. If you are a very busy person but you are dying to add color to your natural hair, without having to dye your hair, colored extensions/weaves are a great alternative. Natural hair can be as easy or as difficult in maintenance for you depending on the condition of your hair. The maintenance of your hair should reflect the amount of time that you have on hand, without having to sacrifice the health of your hair to achieve a certain look.

THE PSYCHOLOGICAL ASPECT OF BLACK HAIR

Hair is very important to many women within the African American community. We use our hair as a reflection of who we are and how we would like the world to see us. Stage hair, relaxed hair, natural hair, extensions and weaves holds vastly different meanings to different women. Some women love to wear stage hair as an everyday look, they may love colorful and voluminous hairstyles. Those who wear relaxed hair may love a sleek look and those with natural hair may love the kinky textured look. Extensions and weaves hold many similarities to one another because additional hair is required to achieve multiple looks; like braids and twists for example. In all shapes, colors, and textures, you will find different tastes in style from woman to woman and sometimes hair becomes more than just a hairstyle and more like "Keeping Up With The Jones".

Once a celebrity wears a certain hairstyle, that hairstyle automatically becomes the "it hair" everyone raves about on websites, videos, and forums. Some women can become so engulfed in the image that hair is attached to, that the best way that they can mirror the beauty of that person, is to wear their hair just like theirs. There is absolutely no problem being inspired by a celebrity's hair, sometimes seeing someone of a similar complexion, even down to a similar face shape and hair color, helps us to visualize how flattering a hairstyle would be on us personally.

The problem with this scenario is only finding confidence in a hairstyle that someone else of beauty has worn. Do you have an imagination? We all do and we should not be afraid to wear our hair how we want even if no one else has ever done it and if no one approves, it does not matter. Who says that light skin girls have to have long curly hair and who told dark skin girls that they should not wear bright hair colors? Sometimes because of our own insecurities, we project it onto others especially, if we personally have not shamelessly explored our creativity through our own hair.

It is common on the internet to see a woman be haughty toward another woman for wearing "cheap weave". Some women will honestly be ridiculed for wearing more affordable options because the hair is not "virgin" or "remy". It is sickening to see another woman discourage another woman because of her hair. Beautiful hair is beautiful hair no matter what the price of it is. Of course certain kinds of extensions and weaves have a longer life span than others but your imagination might have limits if you can't imagine the possibility of achieving a gorgeous look with BSS hair.

BSS Hair: Beauty Supply Store Hair

TO BIG CHOP OR NOT TO BIG CHOP

Top big chop or not to big chop is the question that every new natural can become consumed and overwhelmed by! The thought decision of taking hair cutting shears and cutting off all of your relaxed hair is a very difficult one to approach. What do you do if you barely have new growth? Thoroughly think about your decision to big chop before you thoughtlessly cut off all of your hair. Feel free to take the plunge if you know that you always seem to get in your own way, but the best way is to make this drastic hair decision a comfortable one. Be well informed of your styling options and to have a background of hair care knowledge before big chopping. Some women casually like to big chop to experience a TWA once again with their hair, or to sport a shorter length of hair. Cutting your relaxed hair is mandatory for having healthy natural hair. You can cut off relaxed length a little bit at a time or big chop. Cut off as much relaxed hair as you can, within your scope of comfort. The sooner you cut off all your relaxed hair, the less chance you will endure further hair damage.

TWA: teeny weeny afro. Very short hair, usually not long enough to cover any part of your ears.

Also overtime, the longer your hair becomes, the more weight each strand has so eventually, your hair will begin to elongate. When your hair reaches new lengths, this appears to be that your curl pattern is loosening when it is not. Some women like for their curls to have more of a spring that you would notice at a shorter length of hair so constantly chopping off longer lengths keeps that person happy with their hair. Your hair can still be long and springy with great hair care. Those subtle curl behaviors that you may only notice with your hair, and whether you like that or not, is up to your preference. Everyone does not have the same hair goals so some like short manageable hair, while others want their hair to grow as long as it possibly can, to each its own.

When approaching your big chop, have a plan in place. Know what hair products you will use or experiment with and know what kind of hairstyles you would like to wear. You can rock your short hair as is, manipulate your own hair to take on a patterned look, or wear extensions/weaves until you reach your hair goals. Having a plan of action will make adjusting to your new hair more of an ease. Things will not necessarily be easy, depending on how attached you were with the previous condition of your hair, but it is your responsibility to do what is comfortable for you. Transitioning with your hair may make going natural an easier experience for you. Remember to do what is comfortable, you do not have to make a rash decision, the way that you want to wear your hair is held to your consent.

LISTENING TO YOURSELF AND YOUR HAIR

Truly listening to yourself, even in relation to your hair decisions, is an important facet of who you are as an individual. Since birth we have been conditioned to be conformists. Listening to your higher authority and not questioning them leaves you to think that they obviously know better at something than you do. This train of thought spills over into every aspect of our lives, even as adults, and often, this places us in a comfortable environment of conformity. Going against the grain as a free thinker can be nerving especially if you feel as though you stand alone in that situation. When it comes to your hair, as minuscule as the topic of hair may appear to others, hair is reflective of our image and self-confidence so it is very important that your hair represents you well and no matter how anyone else may feel about your hair, you are secure about it.

How do you want to wear your hair? The answer is simple, while executing your decision can be very difficult, complicated, or not much of a thought! Do you want natural hair? If not or if so, keep asking yourself why until it leads you to the very thing that continues to hold you back or, to your reason as to why you have made your choice. Having natural hair should not be done to prove to anyone that you are truly "unashamed" of yourself. People with extreme views could take something as innocent as wearing a fragrance to say that you are ashamed of the scent that you naturally have, so you use fragrance and soaps to cover up your natural self. If internally, you do not reflect the image that you feel you have within, change it. Life is honestly too short to worry about the opinions of others. To put this all into perspective, many terminally ill patients were interviewed about whether or not they had regrets and there were a few, but everyone commonly regretting one thing. No matter age, race, or religion, they regretted caring about the opinions of others to the point that it held them back from making life decisions that they wanted to make. Honestly, majority of people are afraid of change so when change does occur, it's confusing, unnecessary, and rejected.

To make the best decisions for your hair, listen to what you want, not the opinions of others.

AFTERWORDS

This book was such a joy to write and it is well needed for those seeking knowledge about hair, hair advice, and insight in relation to someone else's personal hair experiences. Sometimes I find myself thinking about the "what if" when it comes to my hair. What if I never had a chemical relaxer, would I have longer hair? How long would my hair be? If I continued to have natural hair growing up, would I start to relax it? If I had the knowledge and experience that I have now, earlier in my life, how great of a story could I tell? Then I acknowledge once again that if things were any different, this book would have not been written.

This book could not have possibly been written if my hair condition was perfected since birth. What would inspire me to help those who struggle if I honestly do not understand their struggle? How can I truly guide someone who is trying to get through a difficult hair situation if I have never had one, or have gone through what they are experiencing exactly? How can I or anyone else be taken seriously without much experience or proof to show?

Before I conceived the foundation of this natural hair care book, I thought, why would anybody want to read this? I have been natural since September 2010, which makes me shy of 3 years natural to date. I also transitioned with weaves and extensions, big chopped, and cut unnecessary length off because of the confusion that I had about elongation. Even with that background, along with going through an extensive amount of trial and error, I viewed my voice as a peep in comparison to someone who has hair that grazes their back.

There are combinations of things within me that make up who I am, that no one can duplicate and the same goes for others. The person with floor length hair has no greater opinion about hair care than I have, they have their success and struggles and so do I. They may not even have the thickest and kinkiest of hair like I do, so how can they relate to someone with a great deal of shrinkage, breakage, or frizz?

Everyone has a story to be told and everyone needs guidance at one point or another in their lives. As you near the end of this book, I want to come to a close with an important message.

A very important aspect of hair was never addressed in this book and that is, the secret to long healthy hair. The quest for this hair will never die and the questions asked by many will never cease. I cannot count how many times someone has asked me how to make their hair grow when I can't make your hair grow. Your hair grows from your scalp without your control, but being able to see your hair reach longer lengths, is the result of your hair regimen and practices. Everyone has a hair regimen whether they purposefully incorporate one or haphazardly use whatever products and tools nearby. A healthy hair care regimen will allow your hair to keep length rather than constantly breaking off as it grows.

There is no secret to long healthy hair and if there was a secret explanation to hair length and growth, someone would tell it or

I would tell it! Think of your hair in relation to weight loss, how long does it take to lose weight? It could take months, years, or a lifetime depending on how much weight you need to lose, your eating habits, and exercise habits. If you eat horrible and barely exercise, it's certain that you will gain weight instead of lose weight. It takes dedication to doing what's right all the time to achieve the results you want to see. Every day you have to be conscious of the quality of your calories, how many calories you consume, and how often you need to exercise. As you may already know, there is no fix it pill, body wrap, or mind tricks that will get the weight off and keep it off. In relation to seeing successful results with your hair, you have to consistently do what is right all the time. Some people say "I don't have time to work out every day" or "I'm too busy and I don't have much time to prepare healthy meals" and that is how you will become overweight and/or out of shape. In relation to your hair, if you don't make time each and every day to be conscience of your hair needs, it will be difficult to achieve long healthy hair. Take time to detangle your hair, shampoo and deep condition when necessary, seal your ends, and do protective styles as often as you can to allow your hair to reach longer lengths. Refer to my testimony of my before and after photos of my big chop as motivation. Just by following the commandments outlined in this book and incorporating trims into my hair care regimen, I was able in 6 short months to surpass in hair growth what took me 2 years to achieve previously by implementing a simple trim to my ends. Continue to refer to this book for help with your hair care needs and to receive motivation to keep going on this journey with your hair, good luck!

Thank you for listening to my stories and educating yourself on the 10 Commandments of Natural Black Hair Care.

ADDITIONAL RESOURCES

The Official Website: www.Howtoblackhair.com

The Online Store: www.Howtoblackhair.Spreadshirt.com

Business Email: howtoblackhair.breannarutter@gmail.com

Free Subscription Email: www.eepurl.com/Am3Kb

BlackWomenHair YouTube Channel

www.Youtube.com/BlackWomenHair

HowToBlackHair YouTube Channel

www.Youtube.com/HowToBlackHair

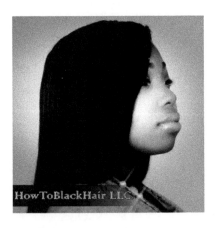

HAIR T-SHIRTS & APPAREL

My Creatively Designed Hair T-Shirts are Available Now!

www.Howtoblackhair.com "Click the Store Tab"

www.Howtoblackhair.Spreadshirt.com

Other Designs, Sweatshirts, Phone Cases, and much more

AVAILABLE as well!

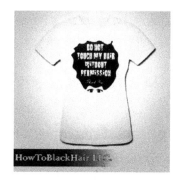

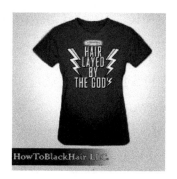

" DO NOT TOUCH MY HAIR "   "HAIR LAYED BY THE GODS"

T-SHIRT   T-SHIRT

DEFINITION GUIDE

THE LOIS HAIR TYPING SYSTEM: *this system identifies the shape of your hair strands with the shape of its letters representing the shape of your strands.*

THE ANDRE WALKER HAIR TYPING SYSTEM: *this system identifies the look of a curl pattern more than the feel and texture of the curl pattern.*

BIG CHOP: *the process of cutting relaxed or permed ends of one's hair when transitioning from chemically processed hair to natural hair.*

DRY HAIR: *hair that lacks the necessary moisture to retain a soft, smooth appearance.*

SINGLE STRAND KNOT (FAIRY KNOT): *the process of a hair strand coiling upon itself and creating a miniature knot on the end of itself; hence a single strand knot. Unraveling them by hand will squander your time, cutting the knots is best.*

SEALING IN MOISTURE: *applying a coating of oil on wet or damp hair to slow down the rate of water evaporation from your hair.*

CO-WASH: *conditioner washing your hair to restore moisture into your hair to combat dryness.*

SPRITZING: *lightly misting your hair when a co -wash is not necessary but, you still need moisture.*

DETANGLE: *to remove tangles, untangle.*

SHAMPOO: *using a cleansing agent to wash your scalp and hair.*

DEEP CONDITION: *using shaft penetrating ingredients to moisturize your hair for a designated amount of time.*

MOISTURIZE: *layering your hair with water, product, and oil to keep hair supple.*

STYLING: *fashioning your hair by manipulation.*

NATURAL HAIR NAZI: *a die-hard natural hair enthusiast that labels others as a true natural based off product choices and/or styling options, beyond the undisputed universal definition of having natural hair.*

NATURAL HAIR: *hair that is not chemically/permanently treated to change the texture/curl pattern that naturally grows from your scalp.*

TRACTION ALOPECIA: *traumatic (or repeated) stress (outside forces) on your hair and scalp that leads to hair loss. This can be seen in the form of a bald patch/patches or a receding hairline.*

WEAVE-A-HOLIC: *an extension/weave obsessed individual that loves to wear many different kinds of textures and curl patterns. It is typical for this individual to constantly change the look of their hair.*

LEAVE OUT: *leaving out a section of your real hair to conceal the bind/attachment of your weave and or extensions.*

CREAMY CRACK: *The slang name/term for a chemical relaxer.*

PROTECTIVE STYLE: *a hairstyle that requires low manipulation with usually concealed ends. It is also free of harsh chemicals and heat. The degree of what is a protective style or not, varies from person to person. For example, two strand twists would be valued as a protective style and not a twist out even though, both styles fit this very description.*

BSS HAIR: *Beauty Supply Store Hair.*

TWA: *teeny weeny afro. Very short hair, usually not long enough to cover any part of your ears.*

ELASTICITY: *hair that can slightly snap back and return to its original shape after it has been stretched or compressed.*

ESSENTIAL OIL: *natural oil typically obtained by distillation and having the characteristic fragrance of the plant or another source.*

HUMECTANT: *a substance that retains or preserves moisture.*

KANEKALON HAIR: *a form of synthetic extension hair predominately used for braids and twists.*

REMY HAIR: *hair taken directly from the head of a donor and gathered with all cuticles aligned in the same direction as it grows from the head.*

TRACK: *bulk hair that is held together in a thin row bound by thread. Also referred to as weave, track hair, or weave hair.*

INDEX

A

ABSORBENCY: *8*

ABSORBENT: *38*

ABSORBS: *10, 13*

ABSORB: *7, 12, 38, 48*

ACRYLIC YARN: *110*

ADVOCADO: *67, 68*

AFFORDABLE: *9, 77, 133*

AFRICAN AMERICAN: *123, 125, 132*

AFRO: *13, 16, 35, 47, 93, 115, 116, 134, 146*

AFROCENTRIC: *4, 91*

AFROS: *6, 91, 94*

ALTER: *19, 20*

ALTERING: *19, 20*

ALTERNATIVE: *58, 132*

ALTERS: *20*

ALOPECIA: *31, 96, 97, 98, 145*

ANTI RELAXED: *122*

ANDRE WALKER HAIR TYPING SYSTEM: *2, 8, 13, 14, 17, 51, 144*

APPLICATOR: *20, 63, 64, 66, 67, 70*

APPLYING: *20, 50, 51, 80, 81, 82, 84, 130, 144*

ATTACHED: *26, 133, 135*

AU NATUREL: *23*

B

BALD: *11, 12, 97, 145*

BANDED: *51*

BARRETTES: *56*

BARRIER: *11, 53*

BARRIERS: *39*

BEAUTY SUPPLY STORE: 3, *10, 56, 103, 134, 146*

BIBLE: *1, 2, 4*

BIG CHOP: *4, 5, 35, 36, 134 135, 138, 140, 144, 149*

BINDING: *61*

BLACK HAIR: *1, 2, 4, 5, 9, 11, 13, 127, 132, 141*

CREAMY CRACK: *3, 5 12, 24, 122, 123, 146*

CROCHET BRAIDS: *106*

CUCUMBER: *69*

CURL: *III, IV, 1, 2, 6,-9, 18, 20, 21, 25, 39, 45, 71, 102, 111-113, 127-129, 133, 135, 144, 145*

CURL CRUSH: *130*

CURLS: *2, 3, 5, 6, 19, 45, 53, 119, 121, 135*

CURL PATTERN: *1, 2, 4, 7-9, 14-20, 26, 28, 30, 31, 39, 45, 88, 93, 94, 102, 113-117, 118, 135, 144, 145*

CURL PATTERNS: *2, 7, 16, 18, 28, 39, 88, 100, 102, 103, 145*

CURL TYPES: *13*

CURL TYPE: *14*

CURLY: *8, 16, 20, 39, 103, 121, 122, 132*

CURLY HAIR: *20, 133*

CUT: *2, 3, 31-37, 47, 91, 98, 115, 116, 122, 123, 125, 134, 138*

CUTICLES: *65-70, 81, 83, 84, 146*

CUTTING: *32, 34, 35, 37, 47, 61, 123, 124, 126, 134, 144,*

D

DAMAGE: *2, 3, 29, 32, 34, 36, 37, 41, 42, 48, 86, 92, 95, 134*

DAMAGED: *2, 3, 29, 32, 33, 34, 36, 37, 58*

DAMAGED ENDS: *2, 3, 32, 33, 34, 36*

DAMAGING: *48, 95*

DAMP: *50, 81-83, 87, 144*

DAMPENING: *87*

DANDRUFF: *78*

DEEP CONDITION: *4, 35, 50, 51, 60, 62, 65, 66, 67, 78, 79, 80, 82-86, 131, 140, 145*

DEEP CONDITIONED: *51*

DEEP CONDITIONING: *4, 35, 50, 78, 79, 80, 83, 86, 131*

DIET: *3, 37, 40, 41, 91*

DISTILLED WATER: *78*

DRIED: *9, 10, 13-15*

DRIER: 39, 78

DRIEST: *2, 11, 29*

DEFINITION: 5, *85, 87, 93, 144, 145*

DETANGLE: *68-70, 79-84, 86, 105-114, 140, 145*

DETANGLED: *4, 9, 14, 53, 60, 105-114*

DETANGLING: *4, 9, 14, 53, 60, 62, 68, 69, 70-82, 84-87*

DETANGLING CONDITIONER: *60, 62, 68, 69, 70, 80-83*

DRIES: *9, 10, 14, 29*

DRY: *2, 3, 14, 15, 19, 21, 29, 35-42, 46- 53, 83, 84, 867 144*

DRYNESS: *52, 83, 144*

DRY HAIR: 2, *3, 19, 36, 37, 39, 40, 41, 42, 50-52, 87, 144*

E

ECZEMA: *12, 23, 24*

EXTENSIONS: 2-*4, 15-17, 25, 26-28, 32, 46, 47, 48, 53, 56-58, 90-103, 108, 118, 135, 138, 146*

F

FOLLICLES: *31*

FUSION: *102*

FRIZZ: *10-13, 85, 89, 94, 151*

FRIZZY: *13, 94*

G

GEL: *61, 72-74, 81, 84, 84, 81, 86, 87*

GLYCERIN: *11, 12, 59, 60, 63, 65, 74, 152*

GRAPE SEED OIL: *12, 60, 63, 65, 74, 103*

GREASY: *6, 13*

H

HAIR ACCESSORIES: *13*

HAIR CARE PRODUCT: *2-4, 13, 18, 57, 58, 72, 75, 77, 95, 123*

HAIR CARE ROUTINE: *3, 14, 79*

ROOTS: *8, 9, 12, 19, 23, 25, 34-36, 39, 45, 67, 80-83, 121, 128, 131*

S

SCALP: *12, 23, 25, 26, 28, 31, 39, 53, 78, 81, 82, 88, 93, 96, 97, 98, 105, 106, 107, 109, 110, 127, 139, 145, 146*

SEAL: 11, *13, 39, 50, 51, 85, 110-113, 140, 144, 146*

SEALANTS: *11*

SEBUM: *39*

SERUMS: *8, 11-13*

SHAMPOOING: *4, 49, 78, 79, 80-83, 86*

SHAVE: *12*

SHEA BUTTER: *12, 68, 71, 72*

SHED HAIR: *9, 14*

SHEEN: *10-12*

SHINE: *10-13*

SILICONES: *62*

SILKY: *11, 13, 57*

SOAP: *59, 63, 64, 137*

SPLIT ENDS: *34, 42, 94*

SPONGY: *10, 12, 13, 17*

STRAND: *2, 7-12, 18, 29, 30, 31, 34, 38-42, 44, 46-48, 51, 80-84, 88, 105, 109, 110, 127, 129, 131, 134, 144, 146*

STYLING: *4, 11, 12, 23, 38, 61, 62, 75, 78-80, 85, 87, 93, 100, 98, 101, 103, 104, 119, 133*

STYLED: *VIII, 10, 102*

STYLES: *3, 8, 9, 11, 13, 26, 34, 47, 54, 92, 93, 102, 118, 130, 131, 139, 134, 145, 155, 156*

SWIMMING: *2, 3, 44, 45, 46, 47-53,*

T

TEA TREE OIL: *13, 60*

TENSION: *13, 18*

TEXTURIZER: *1, 2, 2, 22*

TEXTURE: *8-14, 17, 18, 19, 30, 39, 41, 42, 56, 57, 88, 93, 102, 114, 116-118, 122*

THREADY: *10, 11*

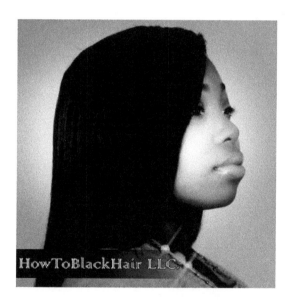

HowToBlackHair LLC.